REVOLUTION
IN FAT LOSS™

HCG 750+ Diet™

Lose Weight and Keep it Off without Starving Yourself.
Easy to Follow Diet with Amazing Results
Recipes, Nutrition Information and Food Journal

Anil M. Patel, M.D.

HEALTHY EATING IS HEALTHY LIVING ™

Dr. Anil M. Patel, M.D.

Board Certified: American Academy of Family Medicine
Subspecialty: Weight Management and Aesthetic Medicine
Clinical Research: Sub-Investigator
Adjunct Assistant Professor:
Touro University Nevada School of Osteopathic Medicine

Author of following Books:

- Instant Access Wards
- Instant Access Hospital Admissions
- Instant Access Orthopedics and Sports Medicine
- Instant Access EKG interpretations and Cardiac studies
- Revolution in Fat Loss: Patel Proprietary Diet

Editors and Contributors:

Dr. Phil Ornstein
Michele Stratton

To find more information about our services and products please visit:
www.iHealthRevolution.com or Scan QR code

Please consult a Physician or medical provider prior to starting this diet.
This book can not be resold, redistributed, broadcasted or reproduced in any way without prior permission.

Revolution in Fat Loss, HCG 750+ Diet
First Published 2011
Library of Congress Cataloging-in Publication Data
Patel, Anil
ISBN-10 0-9847098-0-0
ISBN-13 9780984709809

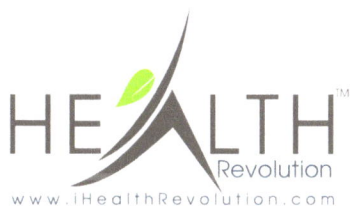

HE LTH™
Revolution
www.iHealthRevolution.com

This book is dedicated to everyone who has made Health their priority.

Table of Contents

I wish it was this easy!

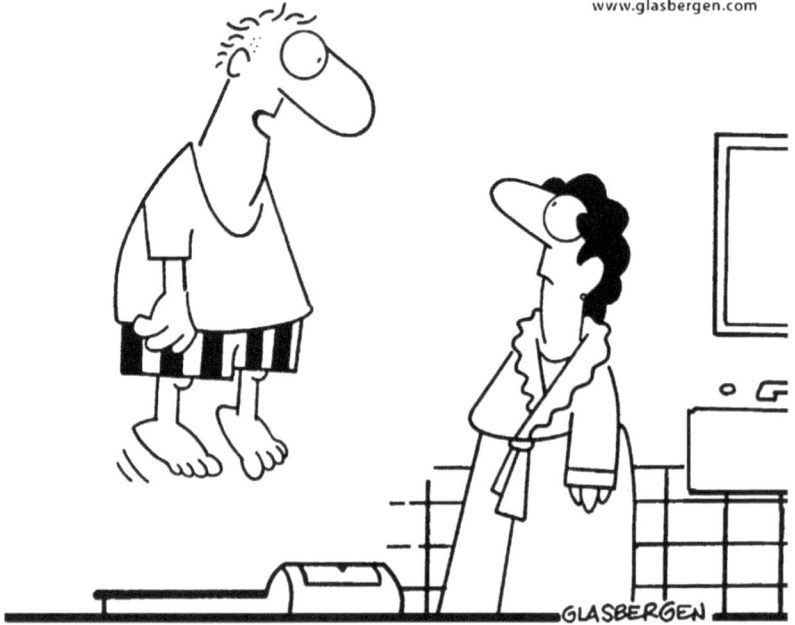

"I lost 198 pounds on the Helium Diet!"

Permission obtained from Randy Glasbergen.

The Purpose and Benefit of this Book

The purpose of this book is to help you in becoming healthy. Weight management is at the core of good health.

This weight loss program will guide you to using natural foods and ingredients.

This book will take you through the process of losing fat without the stress of being on a diet. I have designed this booklet to be very practical and at the same time give you optimal results.

Please consult your physician prior to starting the HCG 750+ Diet™

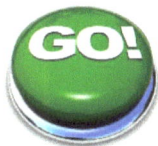

Getting Started

Once you have decided to start the HCG 750+ Diet™, you have taken the first step to a healthy life and minimized the potentially serious medical problems associated with obesity such as cancer, heart attack, stroke, kidney disease and more.

The HCG 750+ diet™ has been designed through intense research by my colleagues and myself.

I would like to be the first one to congratulate you on taking the first step in becoming healthy.

Your journey is more than just weight loss, it is a lifestyle change. This will allow you to continue losing weight even after you have successfully completed the HCG 750+ diet™.

Good Luck!

"The groundwork of all happiness is health."
-Leigh Hunt

Introduction

My story begins in India. Growing up in a town that was comprised of a population of less than 5,000 people, life was rough and tough. Food was considered wealth. You were considered wealthy if you didn't have to worry about food the next day. As I migrated to the US at the age of 12, I slowly tried to learn the English language as well as understand the culture. Growing up in the US I noticed that majority of the people in this country didn't really have to worry about food. I noticed that there were multiple organizations that were open to provide you with a meal. As I matured and finished medical school and started medical training I noticed that there a growing trend in patients I was admitting into the hospital. I admitted patients with heart attack, stroke, pancreatitis secondary to elevated triglycerides, various types of cancers, uncontrolled hypertension, and chronic cellulitis from venous stasis. In the majority of those patients, the condition was due to being overweight. Obesity was slowly creeping into the US culture. It has been over 10 years since I finished medical school and what was thought in medical school about the complications of being overweight is a reality and on the verge of becoming epidemic in the adults. The new trend is even scarier because it is projected that in less than 10 years obesity will be epidemic in children as well. It is also projected that the "next generation" (individuals born between 1990 and 2000) will have a shorter life than their parents unless they really change their lifestyle. This defies human evolution and it is all due to the current lifestyle. This phenomenon is very unusual because ever since humans have been evolving, each new generation tends to live longer than its ancestors. The U.S.A. is not the only country where this trend has been noticed. The data from other industrialized nations has also been following the trend that we are seeing here in the US.

What are the culprits of the upcoming obesity epidemic in the US? There are multiple variables to this phenomenon. First and foremost, we ourselves are to blame for this trend. We as a society have created this culture in which having processed food has become a norm. Having a burger and fries or hot dog and soda for lunch has become a part of lifestyle. Even the places where we are taught about nutrition and health (i.e. school) serve highly processed foods such as pizza, chocolate milk filled with high fructose corn syrup and have placed vending machines that dispense soda and fruit juices filled with unhealthy sugars. The end product of processed food is unhealthy for all individuals. For example, a processed burger starts with steroid-injected and antibiotic-fed cattle and ends with meat dipped in ammonia. Ammonia is used to kill the bacteria but is toxic to humans if ingested. It is ingredients like steroids, antibiotics, ammonia and high fructose corn syrup that lead to a majority of the medical conditions that stem from obesity.

How do you manage obesity? There are no easy answers to that question. There are multiple factors that need to be sorted out. The first and foremost is to rule-out any contributing medical conditions. There are many conditions, such as tumors, and medications that can lead to obesity. Some common conditions are Hypothyroidism, Cushing's syndrome, Depression, Prader-Willi syndrome, and polycystic ovarian syndrome. Once the medical conditions have been ruled out then the next step is to find a diet that you feel comfortable following and will allow you to maintain the weight loss that you have obtained.

As humans we like to see quick results. This is not always a good thing because there are multiple programs that are on the market that will allow you to lose weight very quickly, but to maintain the weight loss you must change your lifestyle. Unless you change your habits you will gain the weight back within several months to a year.

What makes this diet different from other diets on the market? Well, this diet is not just about losing fat. It is also about making changes with your lifestyle. This book teaches you what good habits you should follow and what habits you should eliminate from your daily routine. For example, one of the recommendations that I make in this book is never to skip a meal. In layman's terms, when you skip a meal, your body feels that you are starving. The next meal you have, your body will try to hold on to all the fat and this will lead to weight gain.

In summary, losing and maintaining weight loss is about lifestyle changes, not an easy task but you will appreciate the benefits of a new, healthier you.

Get rid of the unhealthy habits and join us in the revolution of shedding fat and conquering obesity.

What are the causes of obesity?

Obesity is a complex subject and there are a lot of theories out there. Some are supported by science and some are not. I will only talk about the theories that are supported by science.

There are multiple medical conditions that can lead to obesity:

1. Hypothyroidism
2. Cushing's syndrome
3. Prader-Willi syndrome
4. Depression
5. Polycystic ovarian syndrome

There are various medications that can cause weight gain or may interfere with fat loss.

1. Prednisone
2. Any type of steroids
3. Certain anti-depressants
4. Certain oral contraceptives
5. Diabeta and Diabinese
6. Nexium and Prevacid

The theories well respected in the medical communities are: genetics, emotions, human factors (over-eating, eating processed foods, and lack of exercise), and low metabolism (aging process, skipping meals).

1. Genetic factors: The geneticists have identified a variant of the fat mass and obesity associated (FTO) gene which causes one to gain weight and puts one at risk for obesity. This gene has also been linked to Alzheimer's. People who carry the specific DNA sequence are heavier on the average, and their waist circumference is a half inch to an inch bigger. A UCLA professor of neurology, Paul Thompson, states that "carriers of the risk gene can exercise and eat healthily to resist both obesity and brain decline".
2. Emotional factors: Humans are full of emotions. Being in a stressed/ high pressure environment can lead to various types of emotions from

depression to anger. This doesn't really mean that obese people tend to be more emotional. This literally means that some overweight individuals tend to process emotions differently and find comfort in food. With these factors, a catalyst such as psychological intervention may be beneficial.

3. Human factors: In industrialized societies these are the biggest factors that influence obesity. Factors such as over eating, eating processed food, and sedentary life style are common reasons.

4. Low metabolism: It is one of the reasons why people tend to gain weight as they age. This normally starts after the age of 30. Another reason for low metabolism is skipping meals. This is why having small frequent meals actually increases your metabolism and may help with fat loss.

"A goal without a plan is just a wish."
-Larry Elder

Success Stories

"I heard about the HCG 750+ Protocol through a friend at my work location. I asked him questions and decided to try it out. It has been a great experience. To date I have lost around 40 lbs. in two months. I feel like a new person physically and mentally. I always seem to have energy to complete tasks quicker and efficiently. I would recommend the Patel HCG 750+ Protocol to anybody that needs help with weight and diet habits."

J. Romero, Las Vegas, NV

"I highly recommend Dr. Patel's HCG weight Loss Program. Not only did I lose 15 pounds in the 21 day program, but I was also able to safely stop taking blood pressure medicine. I am back to my college weight of 185, feel great, and look a bunch younger. As an added bonus, Dr. Patel provided me with a Body Mass Index which evaluates my weight related risk factors. The bottom line is that I am really glad I did the program."

J. Sprecher, Henderson, NV

"Awesome!! I would recommend HCG 750+ Protocol to anyone who is willing to make the commitment to lose weight."

H.R.S, Las Vegas, NV

"I found Dr. Patel through Teachers Health Trust (S.T.O.P.) program. After going through the program I'm feeling better and healthier. I am looking forward to continuing with my new life style. My sister says I'm happy-happy."

E. Galyean, Las Vegas, NV

"The weight loss program has been nothing short of amazing. The program helped me lose the extra pounds I have been carrying for 15+ years and the focus on nutrition will last a life time. Thank you for helping me change my life for the better."

K. Brenner, Las Vegas, NV

"I am a medical doctor who has had a weight problem all my life. I have been on all kind of diets throughout my lifetime. The HCG diet, through Om Medical, is the best and easiest diet I have ever tried. I want to thank Dr. Patel for suggesting and guiding me through this process."

Dr. Ornstein, Las Vegas, NV

Benefits vs. Risks

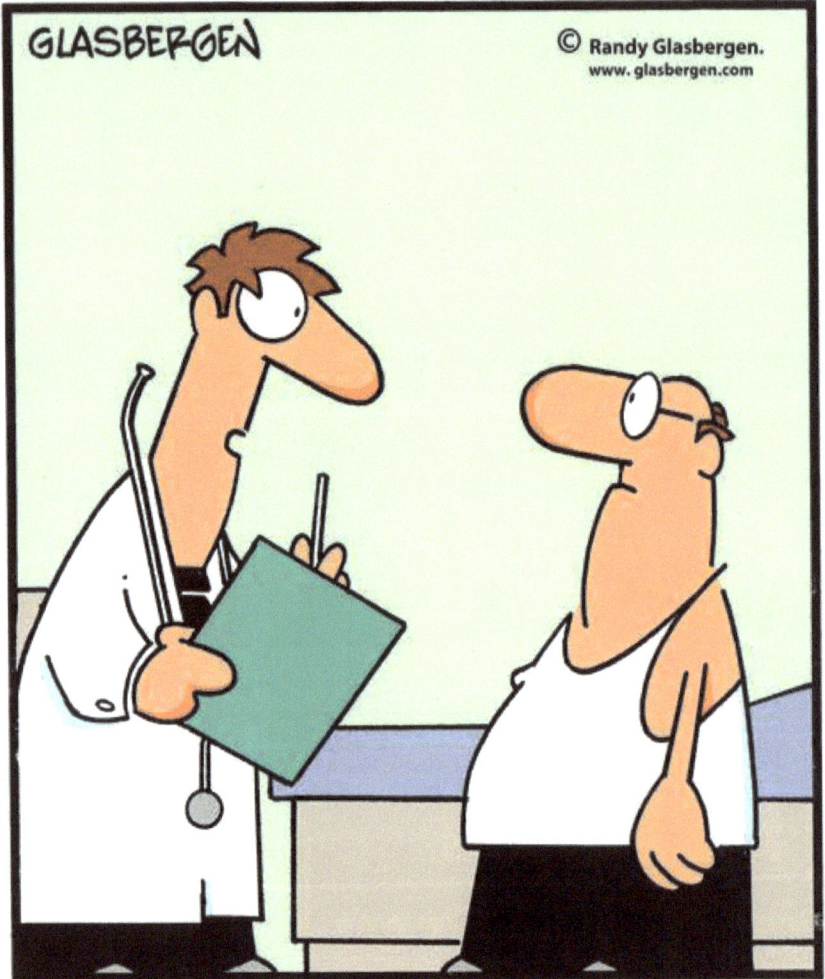

"What fits your busy schedule better, exercising one hour a day or being dead 24 hours a day?"

Permission obtained from Randy Glasbergen.

What you will need to do prior to starting the HCG 750 + diet™?

1.) Read this entire book very carefully.

2.) Keep an open mind about the diet and think positively.

3.) Trash all the items that the book states to avoid.

4.) Purchase a food/weight scale.

5.) Write down your favorite foods and have them during your binge days (first two days of the diet).

6.) Purchase a water bottle/s.

7.) Purchase multivitamins.

8.) Purchase Chia seeds (optional).

9.) Purchase pedometer (optional).

"The first and the best victory is to conquer self."
-Plato

Think Positive!

Believe in yourself!

Tell yourself

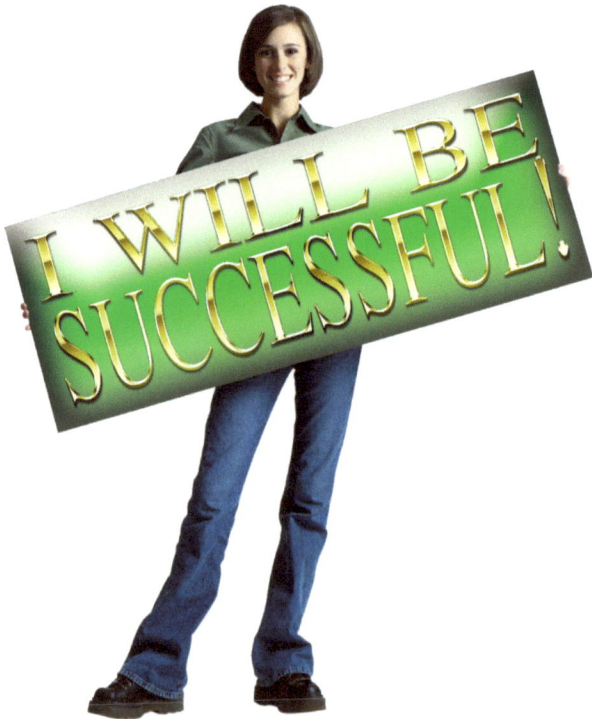

About HCG 750+ Diet ™

The HCG 750+ diet weight loss program was designed after in-depth independent research by our Board Certified Family Medicine Physicians. The protocol has evolved by combining the following elements:

- Low carbohydrate diet.
- Low glycemic index diet.
- Fitness recommendations.
- Food journal.
- Nutritional recommendations.
- Medications.

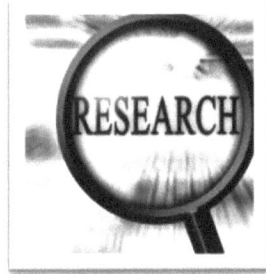

The average weight loss that we have noticed in our practice with individuals who are following the HCG 750+ diet™ is 2-5 lb. per week. We have also noticed that individuals usually lose a greater amount of fat during the first 7-10 days on the diet. A majority of individuals will continue losing fat during the maintenance phase of the diet.

"Put all excuses aside and remember this: YOU are capable."
-Zig Ziglar

Dr. Simeon's vs. Dr. Patel's Protocol

Dr. Simeon's HCG diet protocol	HCG 750+ diet™ protocol
Based on a 500 calorie per day.	Based on a 750 plus calorie per day.
Diet is subject to severe type of food restrictions.	Diet allows for the consumption of a variety of foods.
Diet based on avoiding fatty foods and carbohydrates.	Diet based on the Glycemic Index and low Glycemic Loads and low Carbohydrates.
Avoidance of certain creams, lotions, and oils.	No restrictions on use of creams, lotions, or oils.
Exercising not necessary.	Exercising is required.
Does not use meal replacement.	Specific recommendation for meal replacement with a daily nutritional shake (optional).
No use of high nutritional supplements.	Uses high nutritional natural supplements (Chia seeds).
No food journal provided to track the diet.	Food journal provided to assist in following the recommended diet.
No journal provided to document meals.	Journal provided to document daily meals and exercise.
Recommend patient weigh themselves daily.	Does not recommend that patients weigh themselves daily.

BMI (Body Mass Index) Table

WEIGHT lbs	100	105	110	115	120	125	130	135	140	145	150	155	160	165	170	175	180	185	190	195	200	205	210	215
kgs	45.5	47.7	50.0	52.3	54.5	56.8	59.1	61.4	63.6	65.9	68.2	70.5	72.7	75.0	77.3	79.5	81.8	84.1	86.4	88.6	90.9	93.2	95.5	97.7
HEIGHT in/cm	Underweight						Healthy						Overweight					Obese				Extremely obese		
5'0" - 152.4	19	20	21	22	23	24	25	26	27	28	29	30	31	32	33	34	35	36	37	38	39	40	41	42
5'1" - 154.9	18	19	20	21	22	23	24	25	26	27	28	29	30	31	32	33	34	35	36	36	37	38	39	40
5'2" - 157.4	18	19	20	21	22	22	23	24	25	26	27	28	29	30	31	32	33	33	34	35	36	37	38	39
5'3" - 160.0	17	18	19	20	21	22	23	24	24	25	26	27	28	29	30	31	32	32	33	34	35	36	37	38
5'4" - 162.5	17	18	18	19	20	21	22	23	24	24	25	26	27	28	29	30	31	31	32	33	34	35	36	37
5'5" - 165.1	16	17	18	19	20	20	21	22	23	24	25	25	26	27	28	29	30	30	31	32	33	34	35	35
5'6" - 167.6	16	17	17	18	19	20	21	21	22	23	24	25	25	26	27	28	29	29	30	31	32	33	34	34
5'7" - 170.1	15	16	17	18	18	19	20	21	22	22	23	24	25	25	26	27	28	29	29	30	31	32	33	33
5'8" - 172.7	15	16	16	17	18	19	19	20	21	22	22	23	24	25	25	26	27	28	28	29	30	31	32	32
5'9" - 175.2	14	15	16	17	17	18	19	20	20	21	22	22	23	24	25	25	26	27	28	28	29	30	31	31
5'10" - 177.8	14	15	15	16	17	18	18	19	20	20	21	22	23	23	24	25	25	26	27	28	28	29	30	30
5'11" - 180.3	14	14	15	16	16	17	18	18	19	20	21	21	22	23	23	24	25	25	26	27	28	28	29	30
6'0" - 182.8	13	14	14	15	16	17	17	18	19	19	20	21	21	22	23	23	24	25	25	26	27	27	28	29
6'1" - 185.4	13	13	14	15	15	16	17	17	18	19	19	20	21	21	22	23	23	24	25	25	26	27	27	28
6'2" - 187.9	12	13	14	14	15	16	16	17	18	18	19	19	20	21	21	22	23	23	24	25	25	26	27	27
6'3" - 190.5	12	13	13	14	15	15	16	16	17	18	18	19	20	20	21	21	22	23	23	24	25	25	26	26
6'4" - 193.0	12	12	13	14	14	15	15	16	17	17	18	18	19	20	20	21	22	22	23	23	24	25	25	26

BMI	Weight Status
Below 18.5	Underweight
18.5 – 24.9	Normal
25.0 – 29.9	Overweight
30.0 and Above	Obese

For example, here are the weight ranges, the corresponding BMI ranges, and the weight status categories for a sample height.

Height	Weight Range	BMI	Weight Status
	124 lb. or less	Below 18.5	Underweight
5' 9"	125 lb. to 168 lb.	18.5 to 24.9	Normal
	169 lb. to 202 lb.	25.0 to 29.9	Overweight
	203 lb. or more	30 or higher	Obese

What is BMI?

Body Mass Index (BMI) is a number calculated from a person's weight and height. BMI is a fairly reliable indicator of body fatness for most people. BMI does not measure body fat directly, but research has shown that BMI correlates to direct measures of body fat, such as underwater weighing and dual energy x-ray absorptiometry (DXA).1, 2 BMI can be considered an alternative for direct measures of body fat. Additionally, BMI is an inexpensive and easy-to-perform method of screening for weight categories that may lead to health problems.

How is BMI used?

BMI is used as a screening tool to identify possible weight problems for adults. However, BMI is not a diagnostic tool. For example, a person may have a high BMI. However, to determine if excess weight is a health risk, a healthcare provider would need to perform further assessments. These assessments might include skinfold thickness measurements, evaluations of diet, physical activity, family history, and other appropriate health screenings.

Why does CDC use BMI to measure overweight and obesity?

Calculating BMI is one of the best methods for population assessment of overweight and obesity. Because calculation requires only height and weight, it is inexpensive and easy to use for clinicians and for the general public. The use of BMI allows people to compare their own weight status to that of the general population.

To see the formula based on either kilograms and meters or pounds and inches, visit "How is BMI calculated and interpreted?" (http://www.nhlbisupport. com/bmi/bmicalc.htm)

What are some of the other ways to measure obesity? Why doesn't CDC use those to determine overweight and obesity among the general public?

Other methods to measure body fat include skinfold thickness measurements (with calipers), underwater weighing, bioelectrical impedance, dual-energy x-ray absorptiometry (DXA), and isotope dilution. However, these methods are not always readily available, and they are either expensive or need highly trained personnel. Furthermore, many of these methods can be difficult to standardize across observers or machines, complicating comparisons across studies and time periods.

How is BMI interpreted?

For adults 20 years old and older, BMI is interpreted using standard weight status categories that are the same for all ages and for both men and women. For children and teens, on the other hand, the interpretation of BMI is both age- and sex-specific.

How reliable is BMI as an indicator of body fat percentage?

The correlation between the BMI number and body fat is fairly strong; however the correlation varies by sex, race, and age. These variations include the following examples: 3, 4

- At the same BMI, women tend to have more body fat than men.
- At the same BMI, older people, on average, tend to have more body fat than younger adults.
- Highly trained athletes may have a high BMI because of increased muscularity rather than increased body fat.

It is also important to remember that BMI is only one factor related to the risk for obesity. For assessing someone's likelihood of developing overweight- or obesity-related diseases, the National Heart, Lung, and Blood Institute guidelines recommend looking at two other predictors:

- The individual's waist circumference (because abdominal fat is a predictor of risk for obesity-related diseases).
- Other risk factors the individual has for diseases and conditions associated with obesity (for example, high blood pressure or physical inactivity).

For more information about the assessment of health risk for developing overweight- and obesity-related diseases, visit the following Web pages from the National Heart, Lung, and Blood Institute: http://www.nhlbisupport.com/bmi/bmicalc.htm

- Assessing Your Risk
- Body Mass Index Table
- Clinical Guidelines on the Identification, Evaluation, and Treatment of Overweight and Obese adults

If an athlete or other person with a lot of muscle has a BMI over 25, is that person still considered to be overweight?

According to the BMI weight status categories, anyone with a BMI over 25 would be classified as overweight and anyone with a BMI over 30 would be classified as obese.

It is important to remember, however, that BMI is not a direct measure of body fatness and that BMI is calculated from an individual's weight which includes both muscle and fat. As a result, some individuals may have a high BMI but not have a high percentage of body fat. For example, highly trained athletes may have a high BMI because of increased muscularity rather than increased body fatness. Although some people with a BMI in the overweight range (from 25.0 to 29.9) may not have excess body fat, most people with a BMI in the obese range (equal to or greater than 30) will have increased levels of body fat.

It is also important to remember that weight is only one factor related to risk for disease. If you have questions or concerns about the appropriateness of your weight, you should discuss them with your healthcare provider.

What are the health consequences of overweight and obesity for adults?

The BMI ranges are based on the relationship between body weight and disease and death.5 Overweight and obese individuals are at increased risk for many diseases and health conditions, including the following: [6]

- Hypertension
- Dyslipidemia (for example, high bad cholesterol, low good cholesterol, or high levels of triglycerides)
- Type 2 Diabetes
- Coronary Artery Disease
- Stroke
- Gallbladder Disease

- Osteoarthritis
- Sleep Apnea and Respiratory problems
- Some cancers (endometrial, breast, and colon)
- Fatigue
- Chronic pain

For more information about these and other health problems associated with overweight and obesity, visit Clinical Guidelines on the Identification, Evaluation, and Treatment of Overweight and Obese Adults. http://www. nhlbi.nih.gov/health/prof/heart/index.htm#obesity

Is BMI interpreted the same way for children and teens as it is for adults?

Although the BMI number is calculated the same way for children and adults, the criteria used to interpret the meaning of the BMI number for children and teens are different from those used for adults. For children and teens, BMI age- and sex-specific percentiles are used for two reasons:

- The amount of body fat changes with age.
- The amount of body fat differs between girls and boys.

Because of these factors, the interpretation of BMI is both age- and sex-specific for children and teens. The CDC BMI-for-age growth charts take into account these differences and allow translation of a BMI number into a percentile for a child's sex and age.

For adults, on the other hand, BMI is interpreted through categories that are not dependent on sex or age.

Body fat percentage

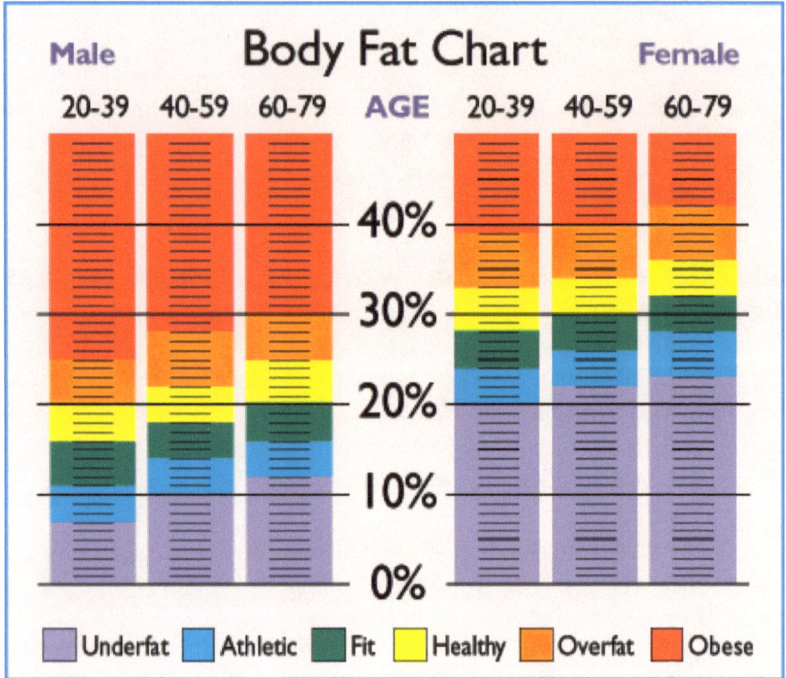

Body Fat Chart

Male			AGE	Female		
20-39	40-59	60-79		20-39	40-59	60-79

40%
30%
20%
10%
0%

Underfat   Athletic   Fit   Healthy   Overfat   Obese

Phases of the Patel HCG 750+ diet™

Phase I: Binge days- Day 1 and 2

Eat as much as you like; Indulge in of all the food that you enjoy.

Phase II: Diet phase

(Must follow the recommended diet).

Must have one option from table A, table B and table C for breakfast, lunch, and dinner.

May have up to 3 snacks in a day

Phase III: Maintenance phase.

(Must follow the maintenance diet).

Foods to avoid with HCG 750 + diet™ protocol

Liquids:

- Alcohol
- Soda/Diet Soda
- Energy drinks

Sugars:

- Artificial sugars
- Product containing high fructose corn syrup
- Sweet & Low
- Sugarcane

Butter

Margarine

Salad dressing

Meat:

- Turkey
- Processed meat

Fruits:

- Banana
- Watermelon
- Mango
- Pineapple
- Kiwi
- Papaya

Fresh corn

Fast food of any type

White rice

Canned food

"Your goals, minus your doubts, equal your reality."
-Ralph Marston

Recommended Exercise During the Weight Loss Journey.

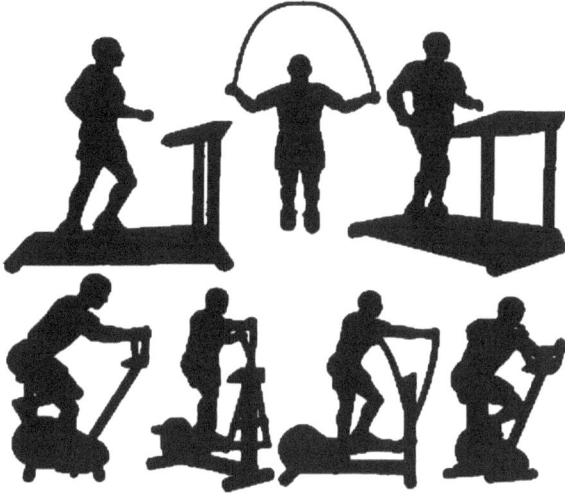

- Treadmill 20-30 Minutes.
- Biking 20-30 Minutes.
- Swimming 20-30 Minutes.
- Running 20-30 Minutes.
- Jogging 20-30 Minutes.
- Elliptical 20-30 Minutes.

- No lifting weights during the medication phase.
- Performing weight-related exercise is recommended during the maintenance phase of the diet.
- NOTE: If your workout consists of greater than 30 minutes, you must increase your protein approximate 20-25% greater than recommended for this diet.

"Put all excuses aside and remember this: YOU are capable."
-Zig Ziglar

"Exercise should be fun, otherwise, you won't be consistent."
-Laura Ramirez

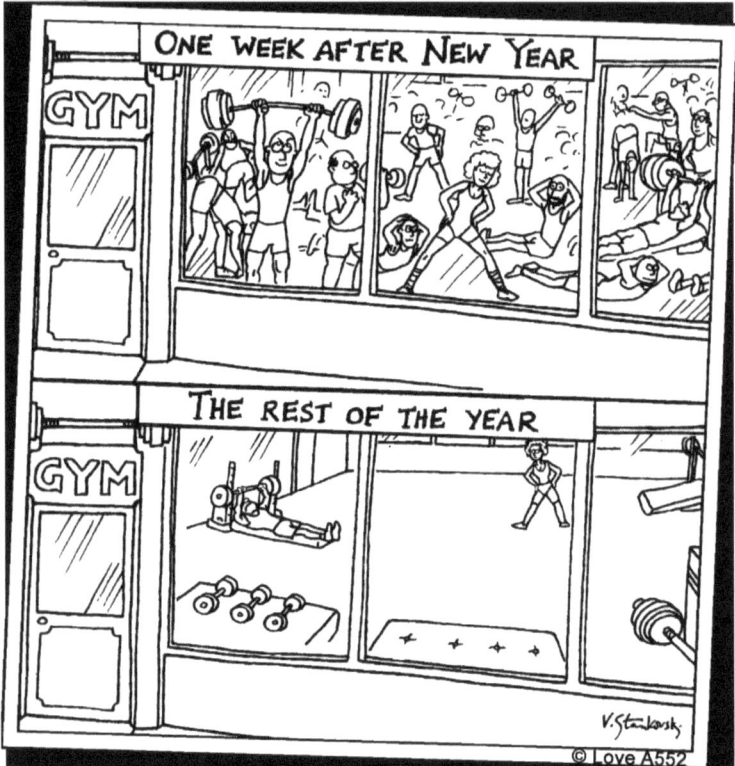

Permission obtained from Jason Love.

Measurement and conversions

- 1c. = 1 Cup

- tsp. = Teaspoon

- tbsp. = Tablespoon

- 1 tablespoon = 3 Teaspoon

- C = Cup

- g = Gram

- 100g = 0.22lb

- 100g = 3.5oz

- 3.5oz = 0.22lb

Important Rules to Follow During the Program.

- DO NOT STRESS ABOUT THIS DIET!!
- For each meal you must have 1 item from A and 1 item from B and 1 item from C.
- You are allowed 3 snacks in 24 hours.
- Avoid skipping any meal.
- ✓ Instead consider meal replacement for breakfast/lunch/dinner or consider healthy granola or breakfast bar for a snack.
- Having 1 snack is mandatory.
- Vary your food for each meal.
- Do not eat the same foods for breakfast everyday.
- Do not eat the same foods for lunch everyday.
- Do not eat the same foods for dinner everyday.
- Do not have any fast food or restaurant food.
- A food item from option A should not be repeated within 48 hours.
- For better appetite control: use Chia seeds (1-2 tablespoons) with each meal.
- Female: Do not take the HCG during your menstrual cycle
- When using Chia seeds- you must drink at least 16 oz. of water with it.
- Constipation: use Chia seeds (2-3 tablespoons per day with 16oz. of water)
- Do not have meal or snacks within 2 hours of prior meal or snack.
- Participate in activities that relieve stress (Yoga, Pilates etc.).
- Get at least 7-8 hours of sleep.
- Consider refraining from nicotine.
- Consider a cardio work-out and avoid using weights.
- Avoid weighing yourself daily (recommend every 7-10days)
- FOLLOW THE DIET AS RECOMMENDED.

"Not to have control over the senses is like sailing in a rudderless ship, bound to break to pieces on coming in contact with the very first rock."
-Mohandas Karamchand Gandhi

This diet may be hazardous to your health.

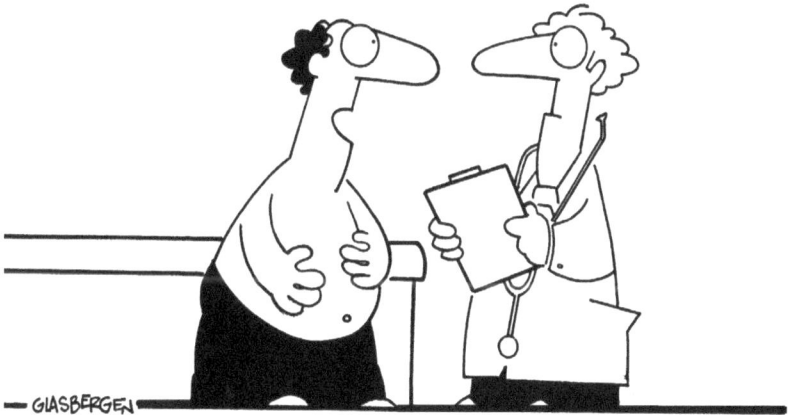

"I'm dieting faithfully. For breakfast I follow the Egg Lovers Diet. At lunch, I switch to the Fast Food Diet. For dinner, I do the Steak-n-Pasta Diet. And during TV I switch to the Chip-n-Dip Diet."

Seasonings / Condiments

Sea salt (1 tsp. in 24 hours)	4-5 Sprays low fat dressing
4-5 Sprays low fat Dijon dressing	1 tbsp. Fajita seasoning (Low sodium)
1 tsp. Light soy sauce (Low sodium)	2 tbsp. Balsamic vinaigrette
Medium onion	2 tbsp. Mustard
Cilantro	1 tsp. Taco seasoning
Lemon/Lime	1 tbsp. Red wine reduction
Red Pepper	Pam Spray (3-6 sprays)
Garlic	4 tsp. olive oil
Ginger	Jalapeno pepper (Fresh)
Black Pepper	2 tsp. Fat-free mayo
Cumin	Saffron
Clove	Sage
Basil	Savory
Cinnamon	Coriander
Bay leaves	Lemon grass
Chives	Dill seed
Cilantro	Ginger
Rosemary	Paprika
Parsley	Nutmeg
Sage	Marjoram
Oregano	Turmeric
Thyme	Mustard seed
Tarragon	Caraway seed
Agave/Truvia/Stevia as sugar substitute (up to 6 packets/24hr)	
Unlimited tea or coffee with only 1 tbsp. of milk	

Snack Options
(allowed up to 3 snacks in 24 hours)

1 c. Plain cereals (No sugar, raisins or marshmallows)
1 c. Chopped celery
1 c. Cucumber
1 Nectarine
1 Orange
1 Apple
5 Strawberries
1 Grapefruit
½ c. Blackberries
½ c. Blueberries
½ c. Cauliflower
½ c. Zucchini
2 c. Alfalfa sprouts
1 tbsp. Hummus
3 c. Lettuce mix with ½ small tomato
2 c. Popcorn (No Salt/Butter)
1 c. Sliced radish
½ c. Rhubarb (diced)
½ c. Chopped broccoli
½ c. Asparagus
2 c. Arugula
3 Prunes
½ c. Raspberries
1 Pear
1 Peach
1 Plum
1 Apricot
1 Clementine
1 c. Loganberry
1 Ugli fruit
6 Almonds (no sugar/salt)

Breakfast Options (must have A + B + C)
A
½ c. Egg white
¼ c. Black beans
½ c. Bell peppers
½ c. Plain Oatmeal
½ c. Mushrooms
1 Whole wheat tortilla
½ c. Cottage cheese (Fat free or Low fat)
½ c. Yogurt (Fat free or Low fat)
1 c. Plain cereals (No sugar, raisins, nuts or marshmallows)
½ c. Milk (Fat free or skim)
B
½ Grapefruit
½ Orange
½ c. Blueberries
½ Nectarine
½ c. Zucchini
1 Small apple
5 Strawberries
50g Spinach
½ Whole wheat tortilla
1½ c. Asparagus (fresh)
1 tbsp. Hummus
¼ c. Mushrooms
1 c. Chopped celery (fresh)
1 c. Cucumber (fresh)
3 Prunes
1 c. Cherries
C
2 Melba toast / 3 Grissini breadstick
2 Strawberries
½ c. Cucumber (fresh)
½ Small Apple
½ c. Chopped celery (fresh)
¼ c. Zucchini
¼ c. Blueberries
¼ c. Raspberries
2 Prunes

Lunch or Dinner Options (must have A + B + C)

A
MEATS
125g Chicken breast
125g Lean steak
125g Top sirloin
125g Lean veal
125g Ground veal
125g Ground beef
125g Pork tenderloin
SEAFOODS
125g Brook
125g Pike
125g Halibut
125g Swordfish
125g Bass
125g Flounder
125g Snapper
125g John Dory
125g Trout
125g Tilapia
125g Sole
125g Mahi Mahi
125g Tuna
125g Salmon
125g Crab meat or Lobster meat
125g Peeled shrimp
VEGETABLES
200g Cabbage
300g Cauliflower
200g Egg Plant
2 c. Okra
¾ c. Lentils (Prefer sprouted)
¾ cup Firm Tofu
1 Veggie Patty (Boca burger)
100g Chick Peas (Garbanzo Beans)
¾ c. Black beans
200g Spinach
¾ c. Quinoa (Rice alternative)

Lunch or Dinner Options (B)

VEGETABLES

150g Spinach

2 c. Green salad mix

1 Large tomato

1 c. Chicory

2 c. Arugula

1 c. Cauliflower

½ c. Chopped broccoli

½ c. Asparagus

½ c. Brussels sprouts

8 pcs. lettuce leaves

1 ½ c. Fennel

2 c. Swiss chard

2 c. alfalfa sprouts (fresh)

½ c. Zucchini

½ Veggie Patty

½ c. Black beans

½ c. Mushrooms

1 c. Snap Beans

100g Green peas

DAIRY

½ c. Fat-free yogurt (Fat free or Low fat)

½ c. Cottage cheese (Fat free or Low fat)

FRUITS

4 Medium strawberries

½ Medium orange

½ Medium nectarine

½ Medium grapefruit

1 Medium apple

1 c. Cherries

½ c. Raspberries

RICE / RICE SUBSTITUTE

¼ c. Quinoa (Rice alternative)

¼ c. Brown rice

BREAD

½ Wheat pita

½ Whole wheat tortilla or 1 Slice whole wheat bread

Lunch or Dinner Options (C)
VEGETABLES
1 c. chopped celery
½ c. Chopped broccoli
1 Medium tomato
1 c. Radish (sliced)
2 c. Arugula
½ c. Asparagus
½ c. Bell peppers
1 c. Sliced cucumbers
½ c. Brussels sprouts
2 c. Alfalfa sprouts
¼ c. Zucchini
1 c. Radish (sliced)
½ c. Snap beans
50g Green peas
DAIRY
¼ c. Fat-free yogurt (Fat-free or Low fat)
¼ c. Cottage cheese (Fat-free or Low fat)
FRUITS
2 Medium strawberries
½ Medium grapefruit
½ Medium orange
½ Medium nectarine
½ Medium apple
½ c. Blackberries
½ c. Blueberries
¼ c. Raspberries
½ c. Cherries
Misc.
¼ c. Black beans
2 Melba toast
2 Grissini bread stick
2 tbsp. Hummus
1 c. Popcorn (No Salt/Butter)

Diet Phase Recipes

Breakfast Burrito

Ingredients
1 whole wheat tortilla
¼ cup- egg white
2 Tbsp.- low fat shredded mozzarella cheese
Crumble bits of bacon

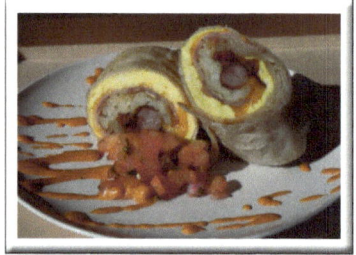

Directions: Spray pan with nonstick vegetable spray, cook bacon per package directions. Remove bacon & set aside. Add eggs to pan. Cook for two minutes over medium heat, remove eggs from pan and spoon onto the tortilla. Sprinkle with cheese and crumbled bits of bacon. Season eggs with salt and pepper. Roll tortilla into burrito. Wrap in a paper towel, and microwave for 10 seconds

Italian Chicken Wraps

Ingredients
3 cups Broccoli (vegetables)
1 cup Bell Peppers, sliced
3.5 oz. Roast/Grill Chicken Breast and slice
Zesty Italian Dressing,
 Fat-Free, 6 sprays
1 Wheat Tortilla Wraps

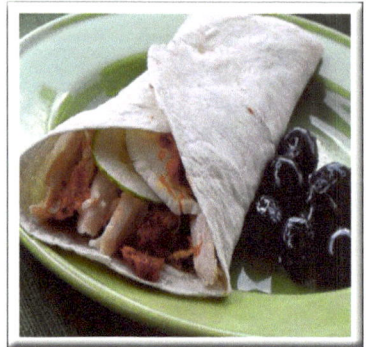

Directions
Sweat veggies with a spray of olive oil and a little water; add chicken and dressing; simmer 5 minutes. Place in middle of wrap and fold burrito style.

Breakfast Omelet Wrap

Ingredients
½ cup egg whites
¼ cup cooked spinach
½ cup fresh Mozzarella cheese
¼ cup diced tomatoes
1 tbsp. diced onion
1 tbsp. diced green or red pepper
1 Morningstar sausage pattie, cooked and crumbled
1 Whole wheat tortilla

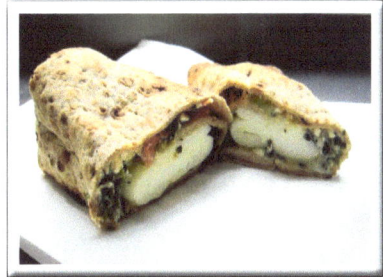

Directions
Mix all ingredients together except tortilla. Place in large microwavable glass bowl. Sauté on (or over) medium heat. When egg substitute puffs up and isn't runny in middle, it is done. Add entire bowl to warm low carb tortilla and wrap up.

Chicken and Mixed Vegetable Quesadillas

Ingredients
3.5oz.   cooked   chicken   breast, shredded
1 Whole wheat tortilla
½ cup chopped onions (red or sweet yellow)
½ cup sliced mushrooms
½ cup sliced roasted red peppers
¼ cup fresh mozzarella

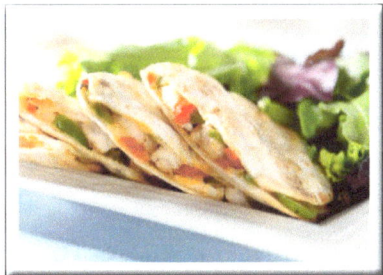

Directions
Coat a large skillet or griddle with cooking spray. Place pan on medium high. Assemble quesadillas, topping ½ of each tortilla with equal amounts of shredded chicken, red peppers, onions, and mushrooms, then fold tortilla over into a half moon shape. Place quesadilla in prepared pan and cook for 3-4 minutes on each side, until golden brown and cheese melts.

Chicken Wrap with Jalapenos

Ingredients

3.5oz. cooked chicken breast, thinly sliced
1 wedge spreadable cheese
1 wedge onion chopped
1 Whole wheat wrap
3 tbsp. Red Hot Buffalo Sauce
2 jalapenos sliced
1 tbsp. olive oil

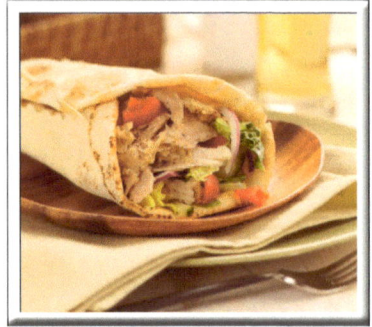

Directions

Heat olive oil in pan and add chicken and onion. Once heated through layer the ingredients in the wrap.

Grilled Chicken Chimichangas

Ingredients

1 Whole wheat tortilla
3.5oz. Chicken tenderloins
½ tsp. Garlic powder
½ tsp. Ground Cumin
1 tsp. Taco Seasoning Mix (low sodiu
½ cup Mozzarella cheese

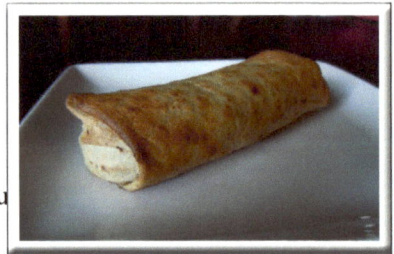

Directions

Grill chicken tenderloins. In a small bowl mix seasonings with 2 sprays of butter. Shred chicken into bowl and stir until well mixed with seasonings. Add about 3 tablespoons of the cheese, blend with chicken and mix well. Split chicken and cheese mixture between the tortillas (down the middle). Roll up tortilla and press in the grill just until crunchy. Top each with ½ of the remaining cheese and melt either in the microwave for 20 seconds or under the broiler briefly.

Vegetable Panini

Ingredients
1 Whole Wheat tortilla.
.65 oz.- Eggplant (strips)
.65 oz.- Zucchini (strips)
3 each- Fresh basil leaves
.25 oz.- Roasted red pepper
2 each- Tomato slices, fresh
.25 oz.- Spinach leaves, fresh

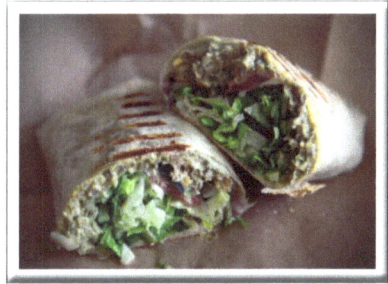

Directions
Grill/Sauté the eggplant & zucchini (season w/ salt & pepper) Take tortilla and lay cooked vegetables in middle and pile on basil, roasted red peppers, tomato slices, and spinach. Fold bottom up, sides in and roll over to close. Place on Panini press or George Forman grill w/ some Pam spray, cook for 2 minutes. Cut in half.

Mushroom Pizza

Ingredients
1 whole wheat flat bread
¼ cup Pizza Sauce
½ cup Mushrooms
0.25 cup fresh Mozzarella (Shredded Cheese)

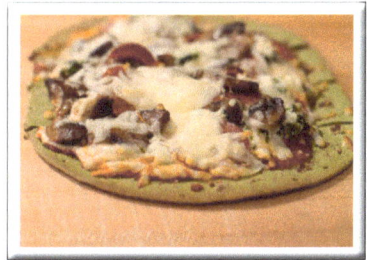

Directions
Place flatbread on baking sheet. Spread the sauce and lay mushrooms on top. Sprinkle cheese and bake for few minutes at 375 degrees. Once out of oven sprinkle over with fresh herbs (parsley, chives, etc.)

"Pastata"

Ingredients

¼ cup Prepared soy meat
¼ cup Boiling water
¼ tsp. Garlic powder
¼ tsp. Onion powder
¼ tsp. Smoked paprika
pinch of sea salt
1 small Portobello mushroom, sliced thinly
8 oz. Shirataki noodles, drained and rinsed
dash hot sauce
2 tbsp. Salsa
2 tbsp. Water
½ tsp. Oregano
½ cup Egg Whites

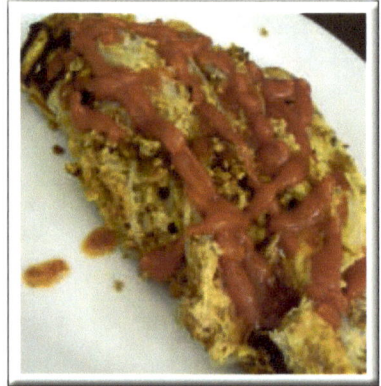

Directions

Place soy meat in a small bowl and pour boiling water and add garlic powder, onion powder, paprika and salt, set aside for 15 minutes. Drain excess liquid. Meanwhile, heat a small, deep non-stick frying pan over high heat and coat with cooking spray. Add mushroom and cook until brown about 5 minutes. Add soy meat, noodles, hot sauce and cook until dry and well incorporated. Spread mixture into one even layer in the pan and reduce heat to medium. Cook for about one minute.

Whisk together salsa, water, oregano, salt, pepper and egg white in a measuring cup or bowl and pour evenly over the noodle mix in the pan. Continue cooking over medium heat until almost completely set, then slide onto a plate.

Low-cal pizza wraps

Ingredients
1 Flat wrap
¼ cup pizza sauce
¼ cup fresh mozzarella
Vegetables of your choosing (peppers,
onions, mushrooms, etc.)

Directions
Spread half the sauce on each wrap,
layer any vegetables (if desired);
sprinkle cheese over both, roll up, and
bake few minutes at 375 or until cheese melts.

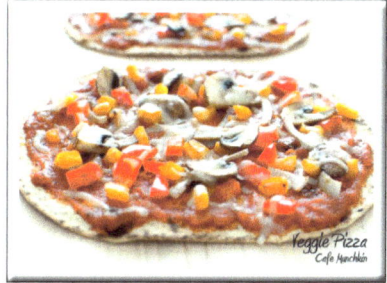

Tofurky, Hickory Smoked Deli Slice Wrap

Ingredients
3 slices, Tofurky, sliced
1- Whole Wheat tortilla
½ C- strips lettuce
2 slices- Tomato, fresh
.75 oz.- Hummus
1 dash of hot sauce (chili powder)

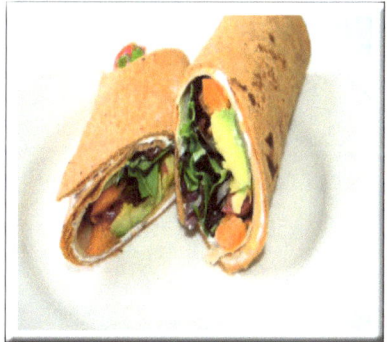

Directions
Lay out tortilla, sprinkle pepper. Spread bottom ½ with hummus and top with
spiced mayo. Place lettuce and tomato on top of hummus spread. Lay Tofurky
slices on top of lettuce and tomato slices. Roll tightly from bottom. Cut in half
to serve

Cabbage stew

Ingredients
0.25 lb. Hamburger meat
½ Med onion (chopped)
¼ Medium cabbage (chopped)
½ cup Tomato (sliced)
Worchestershire Sauce to taste

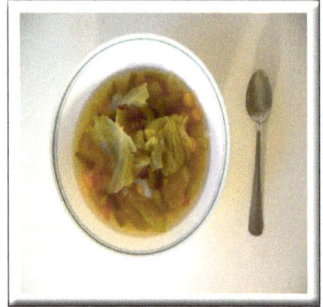

Directions
Boil cabbage in large pot. Brown hamburger meat in a skillet. After it is browned, add onion, worchestershire sauce and tomato soup. Once cabbage is cooked, add it to the hamburger meat mixture and serve warm.

Hearty Black-Eyed Peas

Ingredients
4 oz. dried black-eyed peas
2 cups water
¼ medium onion, chopped
 Pinch of pepper
Pinch of sea salt
0.25lb Ham steak (cut into ½-inch cubes, or 1 ham hock)
1 whole jalapeno pepper (optional)

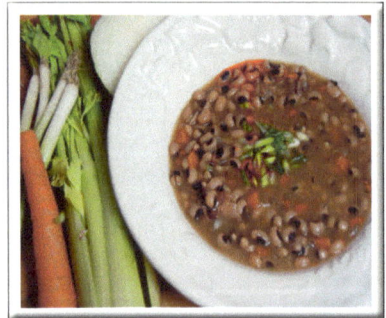

Directions
Bring first 6 ingredients and, if desired, jalapenos to a boil in a Dutch oven; cover, reduce heat, and simmer 1 hour or until peas are tender.

Maintenance Phase of the Patel HCG 750+ diet™ protocol	
Day	**Directions to follow after completion of the HCG.**
1-13	✓ Continue same diet you were on when taking the medication. ✓ Must remain on the same calorie intake and food as on the diet for 13 days.
14-30	✓ Increase calories to (850-1000) ✓ 3-4 meals that include healthy carbohydrates in a week. ✓ Increase cardiovascular exercise to 40 min./day at least 4-5 times per week.
31-60	✓ Increase calories to (1000-1200) ✓ 4-5 meals that include healthy carbohydrates in a week ✓ Increase cardiovascular exercise to 50min/day at least 4-5 times per week.
After 60	✓ Follow your caloric requirement (BMR) ✓ See calculation below.

How to Calculate Daily Caloric Requirement:

- Conversions: 1 inch = 2.54 cm, 1 kilogram = 2.2 lbs.
  Wt. = Weight, Ht. = Height, yr. = Years
- **Men:**
  BMR = 66 + (13.7 X Wt. in kg) + (5 X Ht. in cm)- (6.8 X age in years)
- **Women:**
  BMR = 655 + (9.6 X Wt. in kg) + (1.8 X Ht. in cm)- (4.7 X age in years)

Example:

- You are Male

- You are 42 years old

- You are 5' 6 " tall (167.6 cm)

- You weigh 150 lbs. (68 kilos)

- Your BMR = 66 + 932 + 838- 286 = 1,550 calories/day (Basal rate)

Your caloric requirement will change as per your activity level.

Lightly active (exercise/sports 1-3 days/wk.) = BMR X 1.375

Moderately active (exercise/sports 3-5 days/wk.) = BMR X 1.55

Very active (hard exercise/sports 6-7 days/wk.) = BMR X 1.725

Extremely Active (sports or 2X day training) = BMR X 1.9

Your total daily caloric requirement should consist of:

- 40-50% Carbs
- 25-35% Protein
- 20-30% Fat

Examples of GOOD CARBOHYDRATES	
• Whole wheat	• Wild rice
• Whole oats/oatmeal	• Buckwheat
• Whole-grain corn	• Triticale
• Popcorn	• Bulgur (cracked wheat)
• Brown rice	• Millet
• Whole rye	• Quinoa
• Whole-grain barley	• Sorghum.

Examples of BAD CARBOHYDRATES

- Sodas,
- Candies,
- All pastries,
- Jams and jellies,
- Fruit juices and drinks,
- Refined grains, like white rice,
- Bread and pasta with refined flour,
- Most pudding, custards and other sweets,
- Cakes, cookies and any sweet bakery products.

Incorporating Carbohydrates Into
Diet During Maintenance

How to add whole grains to your diet

- If you enjoy hot cereals, eat old-fashioned or steel-cut oats. If you prefer cold cereal, look for one that lists whole wheat, oats, barley, or other grain first on the ingredient list.
- Eat whole-grain breads for lunch or snacks. Check the label to make sure that whole wheat or other whole grain is the first ingredient listed.
- Eat brown rice or even "newer" grains like bulgur, wheat berries, millet, or hulled barley with your dinner.
    - Choose different varieties of whole wheat pasta. If whole-grain pasta is too chewy for you, choose pastas made with half whole-wheat flour, half white flour and Quinoa.

Important Information to Maintain Your Weight

- Weigh yourself once a week, if you have gained more than 2 pounds, please do a "steak day" that week (See page 66).
- Be cautious of your portion size.
- Do NOT EAT the same food for Breakfast within 48 hrs.
- Do NOT EAT the same food for lunch within 48 hrs.
- Do NOT EAT the same food for Dinner within 48 hrs.
- Do NOT go to sleep within 2 hour of eating.
- Do NOT get less than 7-8 hours of sleep daily.
- Do NOT work greater than 14 hours a day.
- Do participate in activities to relieve stress (i.e. Yoga, Pilates, reading a book, etc...).
- 40-60min. of Cardiovascular exercise 5-7 days a week.
- Refrain from using nicotine.
- Enjoy going out to have "BAD FOOD" (Burger, Pizza, Steak, Fries, etc....) only once a month.
- Do NOT have two restaurant meals in one day.
- If you go out to eat, only eat ½ the portion size (Check calories for food that you are ordering).
- Drink ¾ to 1 gallon of filtered water daily.
- Do NOT skip any meals instead use "Meal Replacement" protein supplement (shake/breakfast bar).
- Limit your carbohydrate to:
  Female: between 180 and 230 grams
  Male: between 200 and 330 grams

"A setback is a setup for a comeback."
-Pastor Bob Lebert

Learn to read labels. Knowledge is Power!

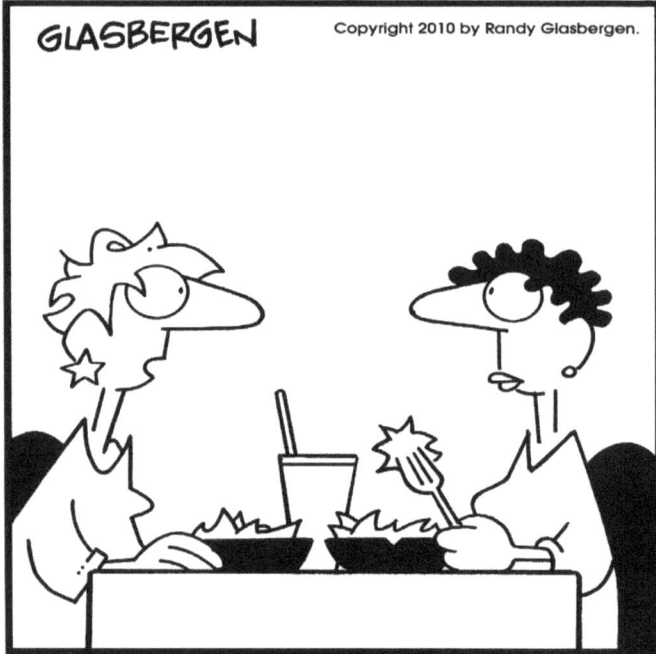

"My husband doesn't know much about nutrition. He thinks 'trans-fat' is a chubby man in a dress."

Recommended Exercise Regimen
During Maintenance

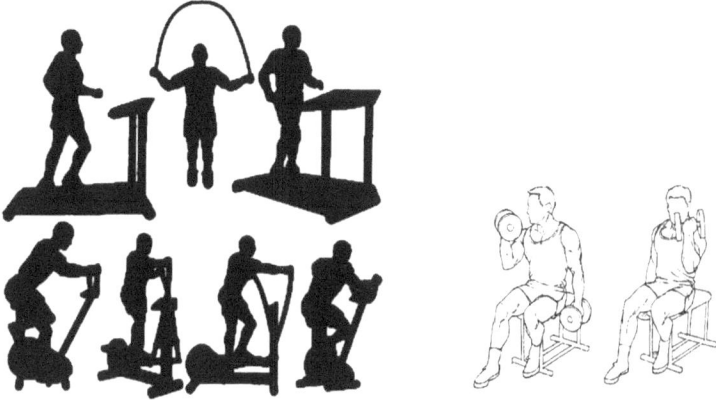

- Recommended 5-7 days per wk.
- Vary your exercise regimen: at least 3 different types in 7 days.
- Young Male: 40% Cardio and 60% Weights.
- Young Female: 60% Cardio and 40% Weights.
- Older Male and Female: 50% Cardio & 50% Weights
- Treadmill 40-60 Minutes.
- Biking 40-60 Minutes.
- Swimming 40-60 Minutes.
- Running 40-60 Minutes.
- Jogging 40-60 Minutes.
- Elliptical 40-60 Minutes.
- Lifting weight 20-30 Minutes.
- Resistance exercises 20-30 Minutes.

Don't let the following happen after working so hard to lose the fat!

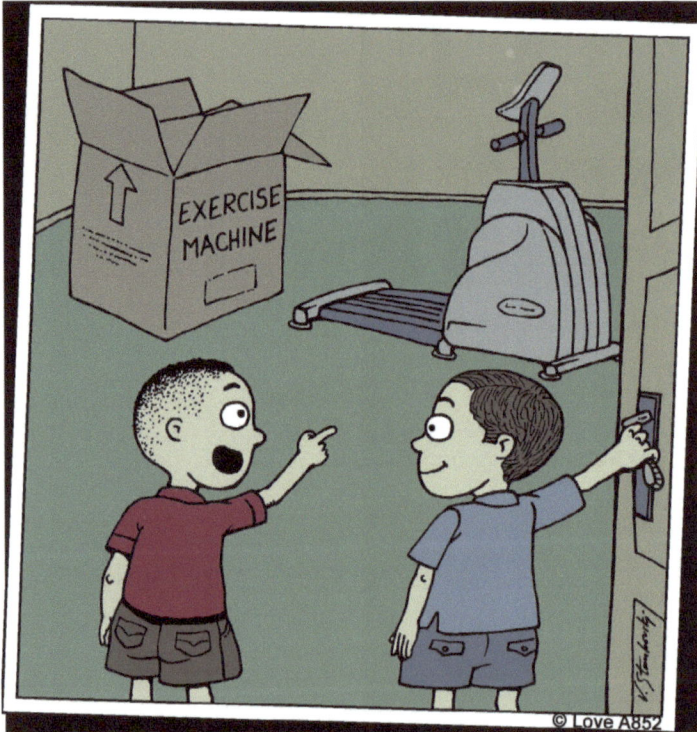

"Hey, we have one of those. You
hang your laundry on it."

Maintenance Phase Recipes

Chicken Salad- made with 3.5 oz. freshly grilled chicken breast, Mustard/light mayo mix (1tbsp.), celery (¼ cup), with sea salt(¼ tsp.) and fresh ground pepper(¼ tsp.)
1 ½ cups = 200 calories

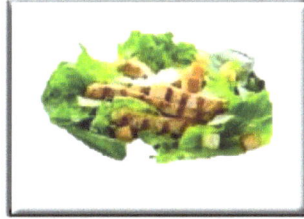

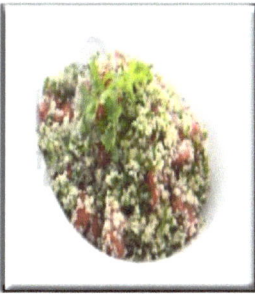

Tabouli- fresh ground cauliflower (½ head) with grilled vegetables (2 cups) salt and pepper (1 tsp.), handful cilantro + herbs and freshly squeezed lemon juice (½ lemon).
2 cups = 65-75 calories

Vegetable Lasagna- thinly sliced eggplant (½ eggplant), zucchini (½), squash (¼), (grilled) lightly covered in marinara sauce (1 cup)
1 cup = 115-125 calories

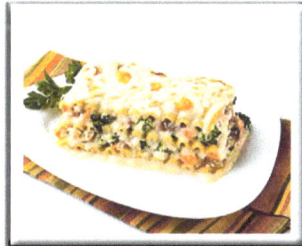

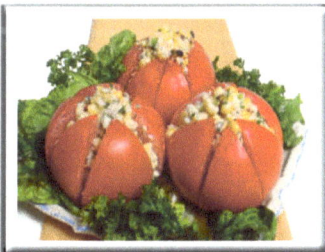

Crab Salad Tomato Bowl
1 large beefsteak tomato
1 tsp. fat free mayo
3.5 oz. Crab meat
Sea salt and pepper as desired
Hollowed out beefsteak tomato, filled with ½ cup of crab salad
1 tomato = 140-150 calories

Mexican Lasagna- lean ground beef (0.25 lbs.), green chilies (2 whole), frozen spinach (1 cup), taco seasoning (1 tbs.), light- enchilada sauce (1cup)
1 cup = 165-180 calories

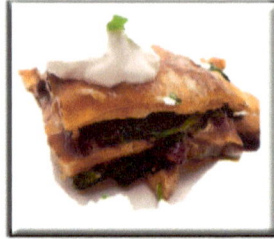

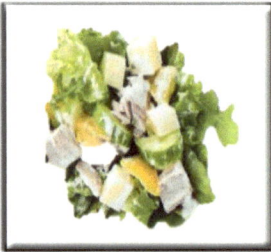

Tuna/Chicken Antipasto Salad- ½ c. kidney beans, 1 bell pepper, ¼ red onion, cucumber with 3.5 oz. of grilled chicken/ tuna
1 ½ cups = 95-110 calories

Stuffed Baked Tomatoes- Roma tomatoes stuffed with ¼ cup mozzarella, fresh basil (2 leaves), sea salt and pepper (½ tsp.)
3 tomatoes = 150-165 calories

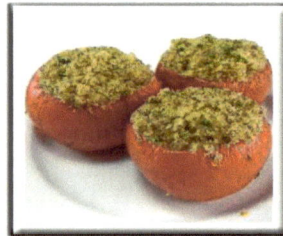

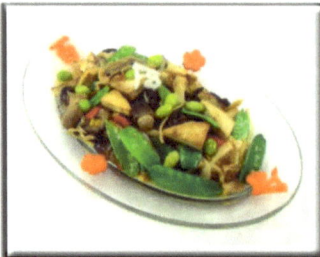

Vegetable Stir Fry- broccoli, snap peas, garlic, red pepper, red onion, shaved carrots sautéed in a soy sauce reduction (¼ cup)
2 cups = 185-200 calories

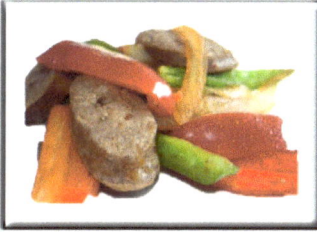

Sausage and peppers- grilled light turkey/chicken sausage, fresh grilled red/green peppers, lightly covered with stewed tomatoes (½ cup)
1 sausage w/ 1 ½ cups of vegetables = 165-175 calories

Herb couscous and Vegetables- whole wheat couscous with reduced sodium vegetable broth, fresh herbs (¼ cup) and grilled vegetables.
1 ½ cup 180-195 calories

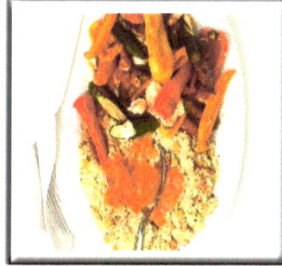

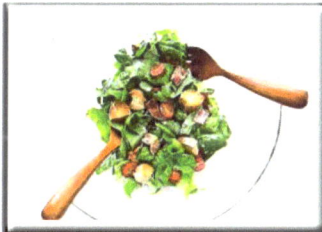

BLT salad- cubed rye bread (1 slice) mixed thoroughly with ½ diced Roma tomato, lettuce (½ cup), mustard/mayo mix (1tbsp.), sea salt, fresh ground pepper (1tsp.) served on a bib lettuce bowl (1 leaf).
½ cup = 235-245 calories

Chicken Pasta Salad- Grilled chicken breast (3.5 oz.), red onion (¼ cup), bell pepper (¼ cup), green beans (¼ cup), bow tie pasta (½ cup), tossed in a light lemon vinaigrette dressing (1 tbsp.)
1 ½ cup = 265-280 calories

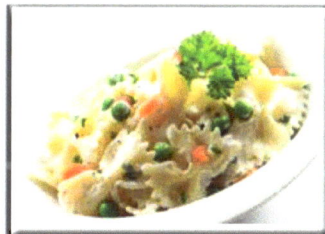

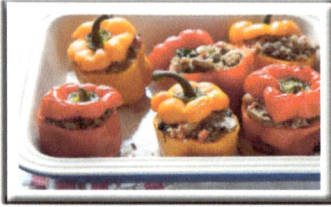

Stuffed Bell Peppers- lean ground beef (½ cup), grilled vegetables (1 cup), brown rice (½ cup) baked.
1 pepper = 255-265 calories

Stuffed Cabbage Rolls- lean ground beef (½ cup), brown rice (½ cup), Mediterranean seasoning (½ tsp.), stewed/crushed tomato (½ cup) baked.
1 roll = 220 calories

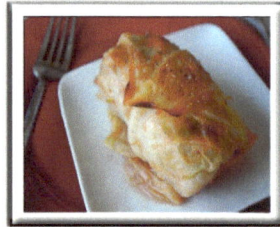

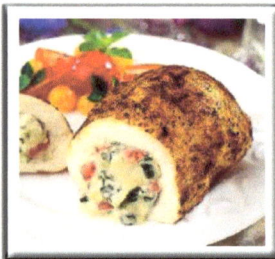

Stuffed Chicken breast- chicken breast baked/grilled (3.5oz) stuffed with feta cheese (¼ cup), kalamata olive (¼ cup), spinach (¼ cup), lemon juice (¼ lemon).
1 breast = 235-255 calories

Vegetarian chili- legumes, stewed tomato, and chili spices
2 cups = 265-285 calories

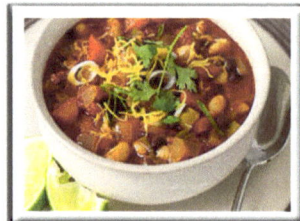

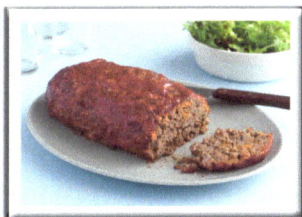

Home made meat loaf- lean ground beef (3.5 oz.), chopped onion (1 half), panko bread crumbs (½ cup), parmesan cheese(¼ cup), seasonings (1 tsp.), stewed tomato (1 cup) baked
2 slices (1 inch)= 260-275 calories

Chili Verde- bell pepper (1 whole), onion (½), garlic (1 clove), chili powder (1 tbs.), cumin (1 tsp.), cayenne (1 tsp.), fresh tomatillo (3 whole), kidney beans (½ cup)
2 cups =265-275 calories

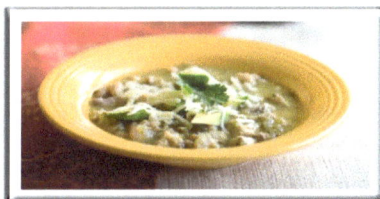

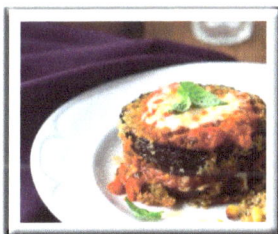

Baked Eggplant parmesan- sliced eggplant dredged in seasoned flour/ Italian bread crumbs (2 cups), marinara sauce (1 cup) baked
2 slices = 290-310 calories

Rustic stew- Diced chicken breast (3.5 oz.), sautéed with scallions (¼ cup), onion (¼ cup), garlic (1 clove), tomato (½ medium), low sodium chicken broth (2 cups), cumin (1 tsp.), lime juice and cilantro (1tbsp.)
2 cups 300-315 calories

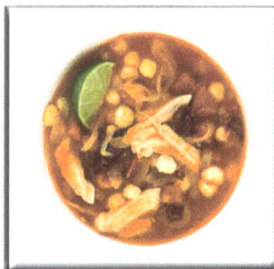

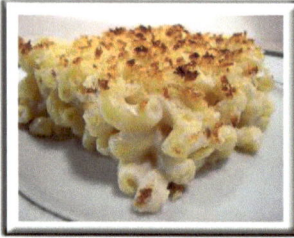

Three Cheese Mac & Cheese- whole wheat pasta (1 cup), parmesan (¼ cup), mozzarella (¼ cup), cheddar(¼ cup), roasted tomato (1 cup)
2 cups = 335-340 calories

Shepherd's Pie- lean ground beef (0.25 lb.), peas (¼ cup), onions (¼ cup), phyllo dough (1 sheet) (no mash) baked
2 cups = 440-455 calories

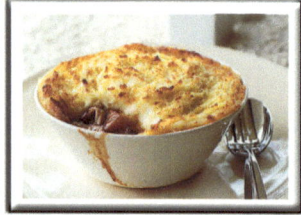

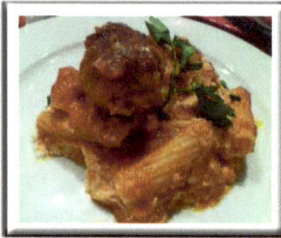

Baked Ziti & Meat balls- whole wheat pasta, lean ground beef meatballs (2 x 2 oz.), light marinara sauce (1 cup)
2 cups = 225-245 calories

Earthy Risotto- Arborio rice, mushrooms (½ cup), parmesan cheese (¼ cup), low sodium chicken stock (1 ½ cup)
2 cups = 420-430 calories

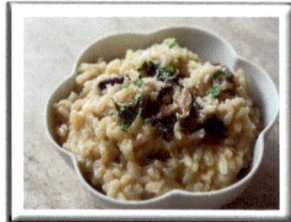

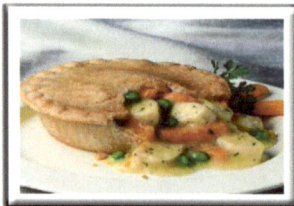

Chicken Pot Pie- grilled chicken (3.5 oz. breast), peas (¼ cup), phyllo dough (1 sheet), reduced sodium chicken stock
2 cups = 385-400 calories

Pasta Primavera- whole wheat pasta, snap peas (¼ cup), green beans (1/4 cup), diced ham (¼ cup), parmesan cheese (1tbsp), lemon juice (¼ lemon)
2 cups =365-380 calories

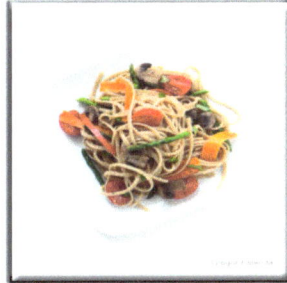

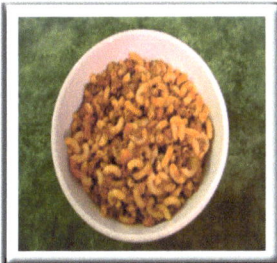

Goulash- whole wheat ziti, stewed tomato (½ cup), lean ground beef
2 cups = 310-320 calories

Saltimbocca- veal (pounded thin) (3.5 oz.) ham, rolled and stuffed with fresh herbs (¼ cup), sautéed in dry white wine/lemon juice (½ cup)
2 rolls = 410-420 calories

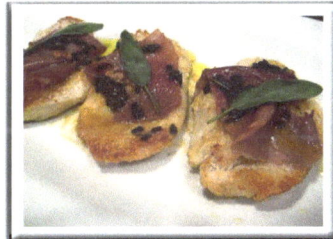

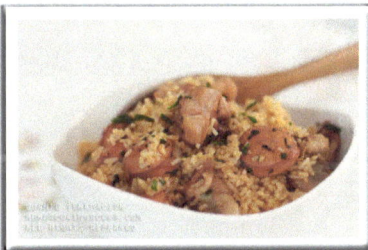

Jambalaya- long grain brown or wild rice (½ cup), chicken stock, lean chicken sausage(½ sausage), fresh vegetables (½ cup), stewed tomato(½ cup)
2 cups=395- 410 calories

Frequently Asked Questions (FAQ)

1. What is HCG and how does it work?

HCG stands for Human Chorionic Gonadotropin.

HCG is a hormone naturally produced in the body. It has many functions and is used medically to treat a variety of conditions. It is the hormone that during pregnancy doubles in amount every two days. This hormone allows the body to mobilize fat and use it as energy for both the mother and fetus. This acts as a "fail-safe" mechanism when energy is needed immediately. For weight loss, we use only a very small amount of HCG to capitalize on this same mechanism. Using HCG in this way does not mimic pregnancy; in fact, it can be safely used by both men and women.

Research suggests that a small, daily dose of HCG when accompanied by a low calorie diet will accelerate the fat loss process.

2. Is HCG safe?

HCG diet is very safe and effective in eliminating fat cells.

The hormone has been in use for weight loss since the 1960's. There have been no adverse events documented by using HCG for weight loss.

3. If HCG works so well for weight loss, why don't pregnant women lose weight?

HCG works to mobilize fat for utilization by the body only when there is a significant decrease in calories. For weight loss, we use a low calorie diet to trigger HCG to help rid the body of fat.

4. Who is a good candidate for using HCG?

HCG can safely be used for those 18 and above.

It is not recommended for those under 18 years of age due to the puberty and the HCG may interfere with the growth spurt.

It is also contraindicated in an individual who has been diagnosed with uncontrolled Hypothyroidism, SLE (Lupus), uncontrolled Diabetes, Rheumatoid Arthritis or most forms of cancer.

5. **Is it possible to be have minimal to no weight loss with HCG?**

   There are approximately 2-3% of the populations who may be resistant to HCG and may lose very little to no weight.

6. **Will my metabolism slow down if I'm on a very low calorie diet?**

   Yes, normally when we cut back our calories and fat intake, our bodies store fat and our metabolisms slow down. This happens because fat is really a life-saving source of stored energy. When a very low calorie diet is used in conjunction with the HCG, the hormone signals the body to use stored fat for energy and eliminates excess fat reserves. It's a natural process, so no ill effects on your metabolism will result.

   The Patel HCG protocol has been designed to increase your metabolism by increasing the frequency of meals and regular cardiovascular exercise.

7. **The HCG diet is very low calorie, will I get hungry?**

   The Patel HCG750+ diet is based on 750+ calories. It is not based on less than 500 calories like the original Dr. Simeon's protocol.

   Because HCG mobilizes fat and makes it available to the body as an energy source, it naturally reduces appetite. So even though you are taking in fewer calories, your body can access the energy you have stored in fat cells. After 3-4 days on the diet many patients notice a significant decrease in their appetite. Overall, most people have plenty of energy and feel good while on the program.

   You will find even tiny servings to be completely satisfying. This is partly due to your hypothalamus adjusting your metabolic rate; but largely due to the amount of calories circulating in your system from the fat being released. It is common that HCG dieters feel as though they are stuffing themselves in order to reach that low calorie limit!

8. Why can I survive on low caloric intake?

HCG causes your hypothalamus to mobilize the stored fat in your body. While you are consuming 750+ calories per day, your hypothalamus is continually releasing an additional 1200- 1400 calories per day of stored fat which your body burns for fuel.

9. What is the hypothalamus?

The hypothalamus gland moderates the thyroid, adrenals, fat storage, and more importantly, your metabolic rate.

10. What is the difference between Homeopathic and prescription grade HCG?

Prescription HCG is usually pure pharmaceutical grade HCG. Prescription HCG can be very effective but must be obtained and monitored only by a licensed medical physician or it is considered against law.

A majority of non-prescription HCG Formula is homeopathically derived and blended with other effective natural ingredients. It does not contain 100% HCG. The Homeopathic HCG itself does not require FDA monitoring, it is recommended that the Homeopathic HCG that is produced by the lab should be an FDA registered lab.

11. Who can be on the HCG Diet?

Anyone over the age of 18 can follow an HCG program. There are no sex or age limits. Men tend to lose more steadily than women. Do not use HCG if you are pregnant or nursing. It is always recommended to consult a physician before beginning any diet or weight loss program.

12. Will HCG interfere with any medications I am currently taking? What about birth control pills or Depo-Provera injections?

The use of Prednisone or any chemotherapeutic agent is not recommended.

HCG does not interact with ANY medications, including birth control pills or Depo-Provera.

13. Will I experience any changes in my menstrual cycle taking HCG?

Because the amount of HCG is so small, there are no changes to your menstrual cycle. Likewise, HCG will not affect your ability to become pregnant, nor will it increase your chances of getting pregnant. You should discontinue HCG while you are on your cycle and start it again when your cycle is finished.

14. Why are some people calling HCG the "Weight Loss Cure"?

HCG is being called the "Weight Loss Cure" because after taking it for weight loss, it reprograms your body to use stored fat for energy when calories are reduced for a period of time. Or put another way, it helps you maintain your weight and not regain the pounds you've lost as long as you maintain healthy lifestyle which includes routine exercise and low fat, low carbohydrate diet.

15. Does the weight loss slow down after the first month?

Many times what we see is a large amount of weight loss in the first 7-10days. You will continue losing fat throughout the program. Typically, inches are being lost continuously while on the program. Weight loss with Patel HCG 750+ diet protocol is achieved in this stair-step fashion.

16. Are there any side effects from using HCG?

There are no serious side effects associated with HCG. Some patients may experience slight headaches, nausea, and vaginal spotting the first few days but this is extremely rare and mild.

A rare side effect of being on long term HCG is hair loss. On occasions if you are losing fat very fast, it may lead to gall stone formation.

Patients who are on blood pressure or diabetes medication need to monitor their condition daily.

17. Is HCG FDA Approved?

HCG is not approved by the FDA for weight loss, but each state medical board holds the right to approve or disapprove its use for weight loss. HCG has been approved by most state boards of medicine for the "off label" (medication used for other reason besides what it was originally discovered for) use as a weight loss medication.

18. What is different about the HCG 750+ Diet™ Protocol from the "original HCG protocol"?

After in depth analysis of Dr. Simeon's protocol, Dr. Patel re-defined the food content by utilizing the glycemic index to the food options. In this way the appetite centers help control the insulin spike that occurs with foods that are high in the glycemic index. Dr. Patel has also increased the calories; and in so doing, the individual will eat 3 meals a day plus up to 3 snacks. The protocol has also incorporated an exercise regimen to accelerate the dissolution of the adipose tissue which will be customized and modified as one progresses in the program. There are also other changes that have been instituted in the HCG 750+ Protocol to obtain optimal results.

19. How much weight will I lose with the HCG 750+ diet™ protocol?

On average, patients lose 2-5 pounds per week. Higher fat loss is usually expected during the first week. Males tend to do better than females and non-smokers tend to do better than smokers.

Please keep in mind that this program will vary from individual to individual based upon different factors, both medical (i.e. hypothyroidism) and non-medical (i.e. stress). The amount of weight loss will vary from person to person but will be substantially greater than most other diet programs that are available today.

20. Will I keep the weight off?

After completing our fat loss programs, you will find your appetite has changed, your eating behavior has changed and your body will, of course, have changed! This is the perfect opportunity to adopt that healthy lifestyle to maintain your weight. Following the diet, there is a three week maintenance period which is the key to keeping the weight off. With your hypothalamus reset, your metabolism will be different and you will be able to eat moderately without feeling the need to over eat.

Common Reasons for Constipation

- Stress of any type.
- Eating foods that are not in the diary.
- Not eating the right portion size as recommended for each meal (under eating).
- Not drinking the amount of water that is recommended (approximate 1 gallon/day).
- Not eating enough fiber in the diet.
- Eating foods that are not in the diet diary.
- Not getting at least 7-8 hours of sleep.
- Drinking liquid that causes dehydration. (coffee, tea, etc…)
- Not performing cardiovascular exercise as recommended.

Solution

- Drink the amount of water that is recommended.
- Do not drink coffee or tea.
- Consider using Powder Fiber supplement (i.e. Metamucil or Citrucel, 2 glasses per day).
- Eat Lunch and Dinner at least 4-5 days out of a week using vegetarian options.
- Make sure you eat recommended portion sizes in the meal, (Do not under-eat or overeat).
- Do not eat foods that are not in the diary.
- Pick up activity to relieve stress (i.e. Yoga, reading…).
- Perform at least 30-35 minutes of cardiovascular exercise.

Common Reasons for Plateau (no weight change in 7 days)

- Body getting used to the eating patterns/calories
- Eating the same food for breakfast.
- Eating the same food for lunch.
- Eating the same food for dinner.
- Stress of any type.
- Eating foods that are not in the diet diary.
- Not participating in any cardiovascular exercise.
- Performing greater than 30 min of cardiovascular exercise and not taking in enough protein.
- Going to sleep within 1 hour of eating.
- Not getting at least 7-8 hours of sleep.
- Working greater than 14 hours a day.

Plateau management

- Have "unhealthy meals" (non-diet food) for 2 days but do not binge then on a 3rd day perform a "steak day", then resume the recommended diet (see steak day below).
- Eat variety of foods every day.
- Limit cardiovascular exercise to 20 minutes per day.
- Drink the amount of water that is recommended.
- Get at least 7-8 hours of sleep at least 5 days a week.
- Pick up activity to relieve stress (i.e. Yoga, reading a book, hiking…).

1) What is a steak day?

Steak day is when you start your day with a normal breakfast and you do not have lunch, dinner or snacks instead, you will have a large steak (6-10oz.) between the hours of lunch and dinner + side dish which consists of handful of vegetables or a large tomato. Approximately 1 gallon of water should be consumed on this day.

"We must accept finite disappointment, but we must never lose infinite hope."
-Martin Luther King, Jr.

Common Reasons for Appetite not being controlled

- Stress of any type.
- Counting calories.
- Skipping meals.
- Eating fast.
- Eating standing up.
- Not having snacks as recommended.
- Eating foods that are not in the diary.
- Not eating the right portion size as recommended for each meal (under-eating).
- Not drinking the amount of water that is recommended.
- Eating foods that are high in glycemic index.
- Not getting at least 8 hours of sleep.
- Staying up until late after dinner.

Solution

- Drink the amount of water that is recommended in the diary.
- Make sure you eat recommended portion size in the meal, (Do not under-eat).
- Eat Slow (at least 10-15 min for breakfast and at least 25-35 minutes for Lunch and Dinner).
- Avoid eating food standing up (Eat sitting down).
- Do NOT eat foods that are not in the diary.
- Consider having 2-3 snacks in a day.
- Pick up activity to relieve stress (i.e. Yoga, reading a book, hiking…).
- Do not count calories for each meal.
- Consider chia seeds (1-2 tablespoons with each meal).
- Consider fiber supplement (at least 10-15grams daily).
- Do not stay up late.
- Do not go to sleep right after eating your meal (give yourself at least 2 hours).

"Rule your mind or it will rule you."
-Horace

Fat Burning Foods:

- Sockeye salmon
- Chilean sea bass
- Herring
- Mackerel
- Lobster
- Trout
- Shrimp
- Scallops
- Crabs
- Mussels
- Pheasant
- Wild turkey
- Top sirloin steak
- Flank steak
- Chuck steak
- Lean hamburger
- London broil
- Elk
- Lean pork
- Eggs
- Goat meat
- Rabbit
- Venison (deer)
- Bison (buffalo)

Importance of Nutritional Supplement

Nutrition is the way that the food people eat nourishes their bodies.

Healthy nutrition means your body is getting all the required nutrients, vitamins, and minerals it needs to work at its optimal capacity. Eating a healthy diet is your main way to get good nutrition.

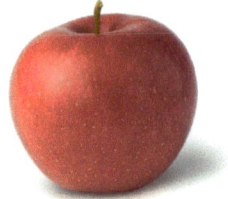

Most people know that a balance of good nutrition and physical activity can help them reach and maintain a healthy weight. But the benefits of good nutrition go beyond weight. Good nutrition can also:

- Improve cardiovascular and other body system functions, mental well-being, thinking process, and wound healing or recovery from illness or injury.
- Reduce the risk for diseases, including heart disease, diabetes, stroke, some cancers, and osteoporosis.
- Increase energy and the body's ability to fight off illness.

Nutrient	Daily values requirement	Unit of measure
Total Fat	65	grams (g)
Saturated fatty acids	<20	grams (g)
Cholesterol	300	milligrams (mg)
Sodium	< 2400	milligrams (mg)
Potassium	3500	milligrams (mg)
Carbohydrate	<300	grams (g)
Fiber	> 25	grams (g)
Protein	0.8 x kg body weight	grams (g)/Kg

Note: When participating in high performance activities, your protein requirement may increase to 1g x kg body weight instead of the 0.8g per kg body weight.

Major protein containing foods:

MEAT/FISH PROTEIN:

Lean Beef, Lean Veal, Chicken, Turkey, Lean Pork loin, Anchovies, Salmon, Halibut, Snapper, Tilapia, Fish eggs, Crab, Lobster, Octopus, and Abalone.

PROTEIN IN GRAINS:

Barley, Brown rice, Buckwheat, Millet, Oatmeal, Rye, Wheat germ, Hard Red wheat, Wild rice

VEGETABLE PROTEIN:

Artichokes, Beets, Broccoli, Brussels sprouts, Cabbage, Cauliflower, Cucumbers, Green peas, Green pepper, Kale, Mushrooms, Mustard green, Onions, Potatoes, Spinach, Turnip greens, Watercress, Yams, Zucchini

PROTEIN IN FRUITS:

Apple, Banana, Grapefruit, Orange, Peach, Pear, Strawberry, Tangerine

PROTEIN IN NUTS AND SEEDS:

Almonds, Cashews, Walnuts, Filberts, Hemp seeds, Peanuts, Pumpkin seeds, Sesame seeds, Sunflower seeds.

Nutritional Daily Requirements

Nutrient	Daily Values	Unit of Measure
Vitamin A	5000	International Unit (IU)
Vitamin C	60	milligrams (mg)
Calcium	1000	milligrams (mg)
Iron	18	milligrams (mg)
Vitamin D	400	International Unit (IU)
Vitamin E	30	International Unit (IU)
Vitamin K	80	micrograms (µg)
Thiamin	1.5	milligrams (mg)
Riboflavin	1.7	milligrams (mg)
Niacin	20	milligrams (mg)
Vitamin B6	2.0	milligrams (mg)
Folate	400	micrograms (µg)
Vitamin B12	6.0	micrograms (µg)
Biotin	300	micrograms (µg)

Nutritional Daily Requirements

Nutrient	Daily Values	Unit of Measure
Pantothenic acid	10	milligrams (mg)
Phosphorus	1000	milligrams (mg)
Iodine	150	micrograms (µg)
Magnesium	400	milligrams (mg)
Zinc	15	milligrams (mg)
Selenium	70	micrograms (µg)
Copper	2.0	milligrams (mg)
Manganese	2.0	milligrams (mg)
Chromium	120	micrograms (µg)
Molybdenum	75	micrograms (µg)
Chloride	3400	milligrams (mg)

Major food sources of vitamins

Vitamin A (retinol)

- Liver, fish, liver oils (very rich sources)
- Kidney, dairy produce
- Eggs, fortified margarine
- Carotene
- Carrots, red palm oil
- Apricots, melon, pumpkin
- Dark green leafy vegetables
- spinach, broccoli, sprouts, etc.

Thiamin

- Whole wheat and whole meal breads
- Wheat germ (richest source) bran
- Yeast, mycoprotein, nuts
- Pork, bacon, yeast extract
- Fortified breakfast cereals
- Oatmeal, potatoes, and peas

Riboflavin

- Liver, kidney (richest sources)
- Milk, yogurt
- Cheese, yeast extract
- Fortified cereals
- Eggs, beef
- Wheat bran
- Mushrooms, wheat germ

Niacin

- Liver, kidneys (richest source)
- Meat, poultry
- Fish
- Brewer's yeast, Marmite

- Peanuts
- bran, pulses
- Whole meal wheat
- Coffee

Vitamin B-6

- Wheat germ and bran
- Potatoes
- Nuts and seeds, peanut butter
- Meat, fatty fish, and offal
- Fortified breakfast cereals
- Banana, avocado, dried fruits
- Vegetables (especially raw), baked beans

Vitamin B-12

- Liver (richest source)
- Kidney
- Sardines, oysters
- Rabbit
- Eggs
- Cheese
- Milk
- Some fortified breakfast cereals

Folate

- Liver (especially chicken)
- Fortified breakfast cereals
- Wheat germ, bran, soya flour
- Black-eye beans (boiled)
- Brussels sprouts, peanuts
- Kidney, other nuts and seeds
- Broccoli, lettuce, peas, etc.
- Whole meal bread, eggs
- Citrus fruits, blackberries, potatoes
- Cheese
- Beef

Vitamin C

- Black currants, guavas
- Rosehip syrup, green peppers
- Oranges, other citrus fruit, strawberries
- Cauliflower, broccoli
- Sprouts, cabbage, watercress
- Potatoes
- Liver and milk

Vitamin D

- Fish liver oils
- Fatty fish (sardines, herring, mackerel, tuna, salmon, pilchards)
- Margarine (fortified)
- Infant milk formulas (fortified)
- Eggs, liver

Vitamin E

- Vegetable oils—wheat germ oil the richest
- Margarines, mayonnaise
- Nuts and seeds

Vitamin K

- Turnip greens
- Broccoli
- Cabbage, lettuce
- Liver

Nutritional value for common foods

BEANS

FOOD	AMOUNT	CALORIES	PROTEIN	CARBS	FAT
Black beans	1/2 cup cooked	113	7.6	20.4	.5
Garbanzo (chickpeas)	1/2 cup cooked	134	7.3	22.5	2.1
Kidney beans	1/2 cup cooked	112	7.6	20.1	.4
Lentil beans	1/2 cup cooked	115	8.9	19.9	.4
Lima beans	1/2 cup cooked	108	7.3	19.6	.4
Navy beans	1/2 cup cooked	129	7.9	24.0	.5
Soybeans (edamame)	1/2 cup cooked	127	11.1	10.0	5.8
Tofu	1/2 cup fresh	94	10.0	2.3	5.9

DAIRY

FOOD	AMOUNT	CALORIES	PROTEIN	CARBS	FAT
Cheddar cheese	1 ounce	114	7.1	.4	9.4
Cottage cheese	1/2 cup	110	14.0	3.1	5.0
Cottage cheese, lowfat	1/2 cup	90	16.0	3.0	1.0
Egg	1 large	75	6.3	0	5.0
Milk, lowfat	1 cup	121	8.1	11.7	4.7
Milk, skim	1 cup	86	8.4	11.8	.4
Muenster cheese	1 ounce	104	6.7	.3	8.5
Swiss cheese	1 ounce	107	8.1	1.0	7.8
Yogurt, lowfat	1 cup	144	11.9	16	3.5
Yogurt, nonfat	1 cup	127	13.0	17.4	.4

FISH

FOOD	AMOUNT	CALORIES	PROTEIN	CARBS	FAT
Anchovies, in water	1 ounce	37	5.8	0	1.4
Halibut	3 ounces	93	17.7	0	2.0
Mackerel	3 ounces	180	15.8	0	11.8
Salmon	3 ounces	121	16.9	0	5.4
Sardines, in water	1 can	130	22.0	0	5.0
Tuna, tongol	1/4 cup	70	16.0	0	0

GRAINS

FOOD	AMOUNT	CALORIES	PROTEIN	CARBS	FAT
Oatmeal, rough cut	1 cup	145	6.0	25.2	2.4
Pancake, buckwheat	1 4" diameter	54	1.8	6.4	2.2
Pancake, whole wheat	1 4" diameter	74	3.4	8.8	3.2
Popcorn, dry	1 cup	54	1.8	10.7	.7
Quinoa, cooked	1/2 cup	115	4.3	21.5	2
Rice, brown, cooked	1/2 cup	108	2.4	22.8	.8
Rye bread	1 slice	56	2.1	12	.3
Whole wheat bread	1 slice	56	2.4	11	.7

POULTRY

FOOD	AMOUNT	CALORIES	PROTEIN	CARBS	FAT
Chicken breast	4 ounces	193	29.3	0	7.6
Chicken, light meat, no skin	4 ounces	196	35.1	0	5.1
Chicken, dark meat, no skin	4 ounces	232	31.0	0	5.1
Turkey, light meat, no skin	4 ounces	178	33.9	0	3.7
Turkey, dark meat, no skin	4 ounces	212	32.4	0	8.2

What is a Chia Seed?

Chia seed is very rich in omega-3 fatty acids, even more so than flax seeds. And it has another advantage over flax: chia is so rich in antioxidants that the seeds don't deteriorate and can be stored for long periods without becoming rancid. And, unlike flax, they do not have to be ground to make their nutrients available to the body.

Chia seeds also provide fiber (25 grams give you 6.9 grams of fiber) as well as calcium, phosphorus, magnesium, iron manganese, copper, niacin, zinc, and molybdenum.

Another advantage: when added to water and allowed to sit for 30 minutes, chia forms a gel. Researchers suggest that this reaction also takes place in the stomach, slowing the process by which digestive enzymes break down carbohydrates and convert them into sugar.

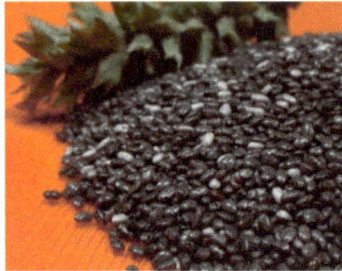

Chia has a nutlike flavor. You can mix seeds in water and add lime or lemon juice and sugar to make a drink known in Mexico and Central America as "Chia fresca." As with ground flax seeds, you can sprinkle ground or whole chia seeds on cereal, in yogurt or salads, eat them as a snack, or grind them and mix them with flour when making muffins or other baked goods. I find them tasty and an interesting addition to my diet. Because of its nutritional value and stability, chia is already being added to a range of foods.

By: Dr. Andrew Weil, M.D.
Source: www.drweil.com

Find a way to focus on the diet

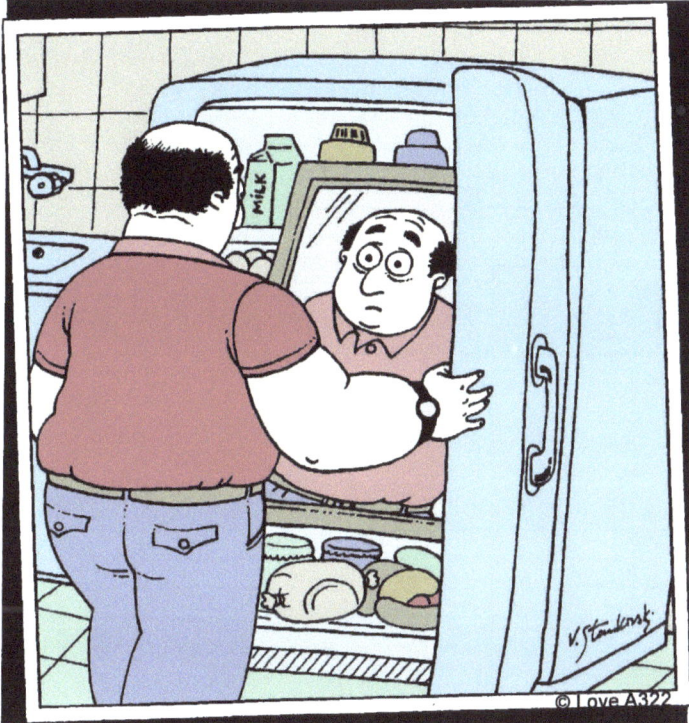

Bob devises the ultimate weight-loss system.

Permission obtained from Jason Love.

DIET JOURNAL LOG

"Where you start is not as important as where you finish." -Zig Ziglar

Daily meal and exercise log		
Day 1 (Binge)	Day 2 (Binge)	Day 3 (Start of diet)
Breakfast Time:	Breakfast Time:	Breakfast Time:
A	A	A
B	B	B
C	C	C
Lunch Time:	Lunch Time:	Lunch Time:
A	A	A
B	B	B
C	C	C
Dinner Time:	Dinner Time:	Dinner Time:
A	A	A
B	B	B
C	C	C
Snacks	Snacks	Snacks
Type of Exercise	Type of Exercise	Type of Exercise
Minutes Done	Minutes Done	Minutes Done
Day 4	Day 5	Day 6
Breakfast Time:	Breakfast Time:	Breakfast Time:
A	A	A
B	B	B
C	C	C
Lunch Time:	Lunch Time:	Lunch Time:
A	A	A
B	B	B
C	C	C
Dinner Time:	Dinner Time:	Dinner Time:
A	A	A
B	B	B
C	C	C
Snacks	Snacks	Snacks
Type of Exercise	Type of Exercise	Type of Exercise
Minutes Done	Minutes Done	Minutes Done

"If you don't do what's best for your body, you're the one who comes up on the short end." -Julius Erving

Daily meal and exercise log		
Day 7	Day 8	Day 9
Breakfast Time:	Breakfast Time:	Breakfast Time:
A	A	A
B	B	B
C	C	C
Lunch Time:	Lunch Time:	Lunch Time:
A	A	A
B	B	B
C	C	C
Dinner Time:	Dinner Time:	Dinner Time:
A	A	A
B	B	B
C	C	C
Snacks	Snacks	Snacks
Type of Exercise	Type of Exercise	Type of Exercise
Minutes Done	Minutes Done	Minutes Done
Day 10	Day 11	Day 12
Breakfast Time:	Breakfast Time:	Breakfast Time:
A	A	A
B	B	B
C	C	C
Lunch Time:	Lunch Time:	Lunch Time:
A	A	A
B	B	B
C	C	C
Dinner Time:	Dinner Time:	Dinner Time:
A	A	A
B	B	B
C	C	C
Snacks	Snacks	Snacks
Type of Exercise	Type of Exercise	Type of Exercise
Minutes Done	Minutes Done	Minutes Done

"The difference between try and triumph is just a little umph!"
-*Marvin Phillips*

Daily meal and exercise log		
Day 13	**Day 14**	**Day 15**
Breakfast Time:	Breakfast Time:	Breakfast Time:
A	A	A
B	B	B
C	C	C
Lunch Time:	Lunch Time:	Lunch Time:
A	A	A
B	B	B
C	C	C
Dinner Time:	Dinner Time:	Dinner Time:
A	A	A
B	B	B
C	C	C
Snacks	Snacks	Snacks
Type of Exercise	Type of Exercise	Type of Exercise
Minutes Done	Minutes Done	Minutes Done
Day 16	**Day 17**	**Day 18**
Breakfast Time:	Breakfast Time:	Breakfast Time:
A	A	A
B	B	B
C	C	C
Lunch Time:	Lunch Time:	Lunch Time:
A	A	A
B	B	B
C	C	C
Dinner Time:	Dinner Time:	Dinner Time:
A	A	A
B	B	B
C	C	C
Snacks	Snacks	Snacks
Type of Exercise	Type of Exercise	Type of Exercise
Minutes Done	Minutes Done	Minutes Done

Take advantage of those stairs in your busy schedule.

SNAPSHOTS by Jason Love

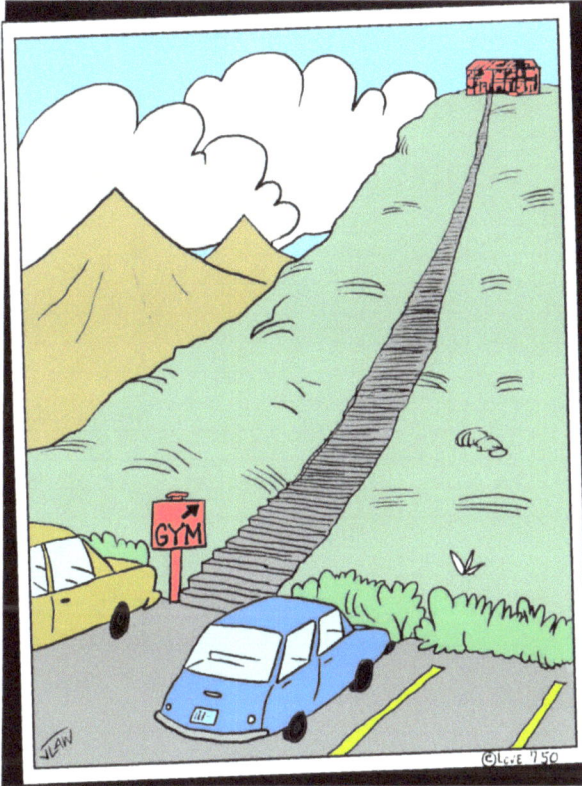

A gym that doesn't *need* Stairmasters.

Permission obtained from Jason Love.

"We can do anything we want as long as we stick to it long enough."
-Helen Keller

Daily meal and exercise log		
Day 19	Day 20	Day 21
Breakfast Time:	Breakfast Time:	Breakfast Time:
A	A	A
B	B	B
C	C	C
Lunch Time:	Lunch Time:	Lunch Time:
A	A	A
B	B	B
C	C	C
Dinner Time:	Dinner Time:	Dinner Time:
A	A	A
B	B	B
C	C	C
Snacks	Snacks	Snacks
Type of Exercise	Type of Exercise	Type of Exercise
Minutes Done	Minutes Done	Minutes Done
Day 22	Day 23	Day 24
Breakfast Time:	Breakfast Time:	Breakfast Time:
A	A	A
B	B	B
C	C	C
Lunch Time:	Lunch Time:	Lunch Time:
A	A	A
B	B	B
C	C	C
Dinner Time:	Dinner Time:	Dinner Time:
A	A	A
B	B	B
C	C	C
Snacks	Snacks	Snacks
Type of Exercise	Type of Exercise	Type of Exercise
Minutes Done	Minutes Done	Minutes Done

"You cannot expect to achieve new goals or move beyond your present circumstances unless you change." *-Les Brown*

Daily meal and exercise log

Day 25	Day 26	Day 27
Breakfast Time:	Breakfast Time:	Breakfast Time:
A	A	A
B	B	B
C	C	C
Lunch Time:	Lunch Time:	Lunch Time:
A	A	A
B	B	B
C	C	C
Dinner Time:	Dinner Time:	Dinner Time:
A	A	A
B	B	B
C	C	C
Snacks	Snacks	Snacks
Type of Exercise	Type of Exercise	Type of Exercise
Minutes Done	Minutes Done	Minutes Done
Day 28	Day 29	Day 30
Breakfast Time:	Breakfast Time:	Breakfast Time:
A	A	A
B	B	B
C	C	C
Lunch Time:	Lunch Time:	Lunch Time:
A	A	A
B	B	B
C	C	C
Dinner Time:	Dinner Time:	Dinner Time:
A	A	A
B	B	B
C	C	C
Snacks	Snacks	Snacks
Type of Exercise	Type of Exercise	Type of Exercise
Minutes Done	Minutes Done	Minutes Done

"If you want to accomplish anything in life, you can't just sit back and hope it will happen. You've got to make it happen." **-Chuck Norris**

Daily meal and exercise log		
Day 31	Day 32	Day 33
Breakfast Time:	Breakfast Time:	Breakfast Time:
A	A	A
B	B	B
C	C	C
Lunch Time:	Lunch Time:	Lunch Time:
A	A	A
B	B	B
C	C	C
Dinner Time:	Dinner Time:	Dinner Time:
A	A	A
B	B	B
C	C	C
Snacks	Snacks	Snacks
Type of Exercise	Type of Exercise	Type of Exercise
Minutes Done	Minutes Done	Minutes Done
Day 34	Day 35	Day 36
Breakfast Time:	Breakfast Time:	Breakfast Time:
A	A	A
B	B	B
C	C	C
Lunch Time:	Lunch Time:	Lunch Time:
A	A	A
B	B	B
C	C	C
Dinner Time:	Dinner Time:	Dinner Time:
A	A	A
B	B	B
C	C	C
Snacks	Snacks	Snacks
Type of Exercise	Type of Exercise	Type of Exercise
Minutes Done	Minutes Done	Minutes Done

"Act as if it were impossible to fail."
-Dorothea Brande

Daily meal and exercise log		
Day 37	**Day 38**	**Day 39**
Breakfast Time:	Breakfast Time:	Breakfast Time:
A	A	A
B	B	B
C	C	C
Lunch Time:	Lunch Time:	Lunch Time:
A	A	A
B	B	B
C	C	C
Dinner Time:	Dinner Time:	Dinner Time:
A	A	A
B	B	B
C	C	C
Snacks	Snacks	Snacks
Type of Exercise	Type of Exercise	Type of Exercise
Minutes Done	Minutes Done	Minutes Done
Day 40	**Day 41**	**Day 42**
Breakfast Time:	Breakfast Time:	Breakfast Time:
A	A	A
B	B	B
C	C	C
Lunch Time:	Lunch Time:	Lunch Time:
A	A	A
B	B	B
C	C	C
Dinner Time:	Dinner Time:	Dinner Time:
A	A	A
B	B	B
C	C	C
Snacks	Snacks	Snacks
Type of Exercise	Type of Exercise	Type of Exercise
Minutes Done	Minutes Done	Minutes Done

"Make the most of yourself, for that is all there is of you."
-Ralph Waldo Emerson

Daily meal and exercise log

Day 43	Day 44	Day 45
Breakfast Time:	Breakfast Time:	Breakfast Time:
A	A	A
B	B	B
C	C	C
Lunch Time:	Lunch Time:	Lunch Time:
A	A	A
B	B	B
C	C	C
Dinner Time:	Dinner Time:	Dinner Time:
A	A	A
B	B	B
C	C	C
Snacks	Snacks	Snacks
Type of Exercise	Type of Exercise	Type of Exercise
Minutes Done	Minutes Done	Minutes Done
Day 46	Day 47	Day 48
Breakfast Time:	Breakfast Time:	Breakfast Time:
A	A	A
B	B	B
C	C	C
Lunch Time:	Lunch Time:	Lunch Time:
A	A	A
B	B	B
C	C	C
Dinner Time:	Dinner Time:	Dinner Time:
A	A	A
B	B	B
C	C	C
Snacks	Snacks	Snacks
Type of Exercise	Type of Exercise	Type of Exercise
Minutes Done	Minutes Done	Minutes Done

"Losing weight will help me gain a new friend. That new friend is me!"
-Unknown

Daily meal and exercise log

Day 49	Day 50	Day 51
Breakfast Time:	Breakfast Time:	Breakfast Time:
A	A	A
B	B	B
C	C	C
Lunch Time:	Lunch Time:	Lunch Time:
A	A	A
B	B	B
C	C	C
Dinner Time:	Dinner Time:	Dinner Time:
A	A	A
B	B	B
C	C	C
Snacks	Snacks	Snacks
Type of Exercise	Type of Exercise	Type of Exercise
Minutes Done	Minutes Done	Minutes Done

Day 52	Day 53	Day 54
Breakfast Time:	Breakfast Time:	Breakfast Time:
A	A	A
B	B	B
C	C	C
Lunch Time:	Lunch Time:	Lunch Time:
A	A	A
B	B	B
C	C	C
Dinner Time:	Dinner Time:	Dinner Time:
A	A	A
B	B	B
C	C	C
Snacks	Snacks	Snacks
Type of Exercise	Type of Exercise	Type of Exercise
Minutes Done	Minutes Done	Minutes Done

"Never, never, never quit."
-Winston Churchill

Daily meal and exercise log

Day 55	Day 56	Day 57
Breakfast Time:	Breakfast Time:	Breakfast Time:
A	A	A
B	B	B
C	C	C
Lunch Time:	Lunch Time:	Lunch Time:
A	A	A
B	B	B
C	C	C
Dinner Time:	Dinner Time:	Dinner Time:
A	A	A
B	B	B
C	C	C
Snacks	Snacks	Snacks
Type of Exercise	Type of Exercise	Type of Exercise
Minutes Done	Minutes Done	Minutes Done
Day 58	Day 59	Day 60
Breakfast Time:	Breakfast Time:	Breakfast Time:
A	A	A
B	B	B
C	C	C
Lunch Time:	Lunch Time:	Lunch Time:
A	A	A
B	B	B
C	C	C
Dinner Time:	Dinner Time:	Dinner Time:
A	A	A
B	B	B
C	C	C
Snacks	Snacks	Snacks
Type of Exercise	Type of Exercise	Type of Exercise
Minutes Done	Minutes Done	Minutes Done

"Victory belongs to the most persevering."
-Napoleon

Daily meal and exercise log

Day 61	Day 62	Day 63
Breakfast Time:	Breakfast Time:	Breakfast Time:
A	A	A
B	B	B
C	C	C
Lunch Time:	Lunch Time:	Lunch Time:
A	A	A
B	B	B
C	C	C
Dinner Time:	Dinner Time:	Dinner Time:
A	A	A
B	B	B
C	C	C
Snacks	Snacks	Snacks
Type of Exercise	Type of Exercise	Type of Exercise
Minutes Done	Minutes Done	Minutes Done

Day 64	Day 65	Day 66
Breakfast Time:	Breakfast Time:	Breakfast Time:
A	A	A
B	B	B
C	C	C
Lunch Time:	Lunch Time:	Lunch Time:
A	A	A
B	B	B
C	C	C
Dinner Time:	Dinner Time:	Dinner Time:
A	A	A
B	B	B
C	C	C
Snacks	Snacks	Snacks
Type of Exercise	Type of Exercise	Type of Exercise
Minutes Done	Minutes Done	Minutes Done

"Take care of your body. It's the only place you have to live."

-Jim Rohn

Daily meal and exercise log

Day 67	Day 68	Day 69
Breakfast Time:	Breakfast Time:	Breakfast Time:
A	A	A
B	B	B
C	C	C
Lunch Time:	Lunch Time:	Lunch Time:
A	A	A
B	B	B
C	C	C
Dinner Time:	Dinner Time:	Dinner Time:
A	A	A
B	B	B
C	C	C
Snacks	Snacks	Snacks
Type of Exercise	Type of Exercise	Type of Exercise
Minutes Done	Minutes Done	Minutes Done

Day 70	Day 71	Day 72
Breakfast Time:	Breakfast Time:	Breakfast Time:
A	A	A
B	B	B
C	C	C
Lunch Time:	Lunch Time:	Lunch Time:
A	A	A
B	B	B
C	C	C
Dinner Time:	Dinner Time:	Dinner Time:
A	A	A
B	B	B
C	C	C
Snacks	Snacks	Snacks
Type of Exercise	Type of Exercise	Type of Exercise
Minutes Done	Minutes Done	Minutes Done

"Nothing in this world that's worth having comes easy"
-Dr. Kelso from "Scrubs"

Daily meal and exercise log

Day 73	Day 74	Day 75
Breakfast Time:	Breakfast Time:	Breakfast Time:
A	A	A
B	B	B
C	C	C
Lunch Time:	Lunch Time:	Lunch Time:
A	A	A
B	B	B
C	C	C
Dinner Time:	Dinner Time:	Dinner Time:
A	A	A
B	B	B
C	C	C
Snacks	Snacks	Snacks
Type of Exercise	Type of Exercise	Type of Exercise
Minutes Done	Minutes Done	Minutes Done

Day 76	Day 77	Day 78
Breakfast Time:	Breakfast Time:	Breakfast Time:
A	A	A
B	B	B
C	C	C
Lunch Time:	Lunch Time:	Lunch Time:
A	A	A
B	B	B
C	C	C
Dinner Time:	Dinner Time:	Dinner Time:
A	A	A
B	B	B
C	C	C
Snacks	Snacks	Snacks
Type of Exercise	Type of Exercise	Type of Exercise
Minutes Done	Minutes Done	Minutes Done

"There is no "try" only "do."
-Yoda from "Star Wars"

Daily meal and exercise log

Day 79	Day 80	Day 81
Breakfast Time:	Breakfast Time:	Breakfast Time:
A	A	A
B	B	B
C	C	C
Lunch Time:	Lunch Time:	Lunch Time:
A	A	A
B	B	B
C	C	C
Dinner Time:	Dinner Time:	Dinner Time:
A	A	A
B	B	B
C	C	C
Snacks	Snacks	Snacks
Type of Exercise	Type of Exercise	Type of Exercise
Minutes Done	Minutes Done	Minutes Done

Day 82	Day 83	Day 84
Breakfast Time:	Breakfast Time:	Breakfast Time:
A	A	A
B	B	B
C	C	C
Lunch Time:	Lunch Time:	Lunch Time:
A	A	A
B	B	B
C	C	C
Dinner Time:	Dinner Time:	Dinner Time:
A	A	A
B	B	B
C	C	C
Snacks	Snacks	Snacks
Type of Exercise	Type of Exercise	Type of Exercise
Minutes Done	Minutes Done	Minutes Done

"Living a healthy lifestyle will only deprive you of poor health, lethargy, and fat."
-Jill Johnson

Daily meal and exercise log

Day 85	Day 86	Day 87
Breakfast Time:	Breakfast Time:	Breakfast Time:
A	A	A
B	B	B
C	C	C
Lunch Time:	Lunch Time:	Lunch Time:
A	A	A
B	B	B
C	C	C
Dinner Time:	Dinner Time:	Dinner Time:
A	A	A
B	B	B
C	C	C
Snacks	Snacks	Snacks
Type of Exercise	Type of Exercise	Type of Exercise
Minutes Done	Minutes Done	Minutes Done
Day 88	Day 89	Day 90
Breakfast Time:	Breakfast Time:	Breakfast Time:
A	A	A
B	B	B
C	C	C
Lunch Time:	Lunch Time:	Lunch Time:
A	A	A
B	B	B
C	C	C
Dinner Time:	Dinner Time:	Dinner Time:
A	A	A
B	B	B
C	C	C
Snacks	Snacks	Snacks
Type of Exercise	Type of Exercise	Type of Exercise
Minutes Done	Minutes Done	Minutes Done

"There are only 2 choices; make progress or make excuses."
-Ellen Mikesell

Daily meal and exercise log

Day 91	92	93
Breakfast Time:	Breakfast Time:	Breakfast Time:
A	A	A
B	B	B
C	C	C
Lunch Time:	Lunch Time:	Lunch Time:
A	A	A
B	B	B
C	C	C
Dinner Time:	Dinner Time:	Dinner Time:
A	A	A
B	B	B
C	C	C
Snacks	Snacks	Snacks
Type of Exercise	Type of Exercise	Type of Exercise
Minutes Done	Minutes Done	Minutes Done
Day 94	Day 95	Day 96
Breakfast Time:	Breakfast Time:	Breakfast Time:
A	A	A
B	B	B
C	C	C
Lunch Time:	Lunch Time:	Lunch Time:
A	A	A
B	B	B
C	C	C
Dinner Time:	Dinner Time:	Dinner Time:
A	A	A
B	B	B
C	C	C
Snacks	Snacks	Snacks
Type of Exercise	Type of Exercise	Type of Exercise
Minutes Done	Minutes Done	Minutes Done

"To lengthen your life, shorten your meals."
Ancient Proverb

Daily meal and exercise log

Day 97	Day 98	Day 99
Breakfast Time:	Breakfast Time:	Breakfast Time:
A	A	A
B	B	B
C	C	C
Lunch Time:	Lunch Time:	Lunch Time:
A	A	A
B	B	B
C	C	C
Dinner Time:	Dinner Time:	Dinner Time:
A	A	A
B	B	B
C	C	C
Snacks	Snacks	Snacks
Type of Exercise	Type of Exercise	Type of Exercise
Minutes Done	Minutes Done	Minutes Done

Day 100	Day 101	Day 102
Breakfast Time:	Breakfast Time:	Breakfast Time:
A	A	A
B	B	B
C	C	C
Lunch Time:	Lunch Time:	Lunch Time:
A	A	A
B	B	B
C	C	C
Dinner Time:	Dinner Time:	Dinner Time:
A	A	A
B	B	B
C	C	C
Snacks	Snacks	Snacks
Type of Exercise	Type of Exercise	Type of Exercise
Minutes Done	Minutes Done	Minutes Done

Congratulations!

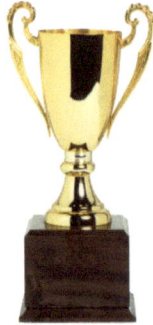

It is not essential to continue logging meals from this point onward but if you feel that it may help you avoid eating unhealthy food then please make your own journal or use our App online.

"Success is the sum of small efforts, repeated day in and day out."
                                                    -Robert Collier

Remember! "Healthy Eating is Healthy Living™"

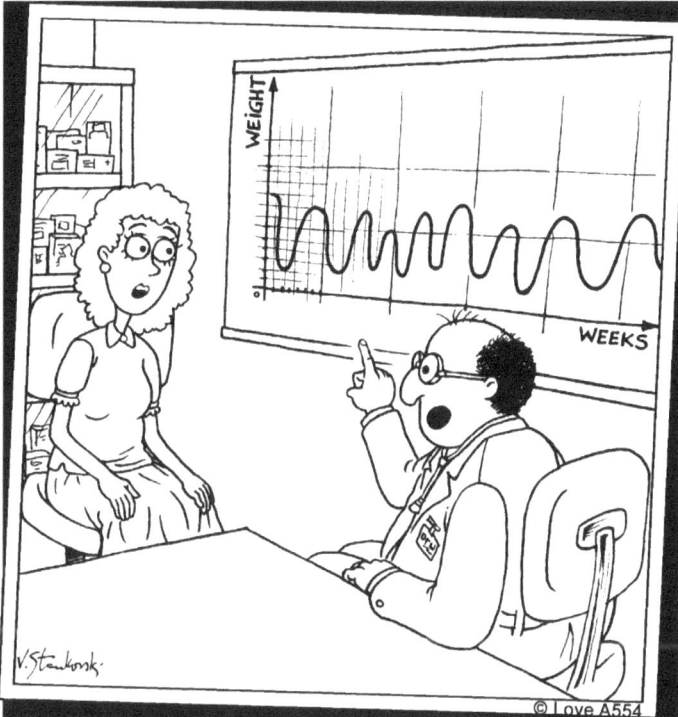

"Congratulations, Kathy. Six Flags would like to model its new roller coaster after your weight chart."

Permission obtained from Jason Love.

Visit: **www.iHealthRevolution.com** to purchase following items:

Scan QR code

HE✦LTHRevolution		
www.iHealthRevolution.com		
Meal Replacement		
☑Advance meal replacement	☑ Omega-3	☑High protein
☑ Daily dose of vitamins	☑ High Fiber	☑ Antioxidants & Calcium
☑ TASTE GREAT!		

HE✦LTHRevolution		
www.iHealthRevolution.com		
Revolution Bar		
☑Advance Snack Bar	☑ Omega-3	☑Antioxidants
☑ Appetite control	☑ High Fiber	☑ Calcium
☑ TASTE GREAT!		
Mobile App.		
	iPhone Android Blackberry

Disclaimer:

In regards to HCG this is the FDA's Statement.

INDICATIONS AND USAGE: HCG has not been demonstrated to be effective adjunctive therapy in the treatment of obesity. There is no substantial evidence that it increases weight loss beyond that resulting from caloric restriction, that it causes a more attractive or "normal" distribution of fat or that it decreases the hunger and discomfort associated with calorie-restricted diets.

Please consult a Physician or your medical provider prior to starting this diet.

STATEMENTS IN THIS BOOK HAVE NOT BEEN EVALUATED BY THE FOOD AND DRUG ADMINISTRATION. THIS PRODUCT IS NOT INTENDED TO DIAGNOSE, TREAT, CURE OR PREVENT ANY DISEASE.

Sources:

1. Mei Z, Grummer-Strawn LM, Pietrobelli A, Goulding A, Goran MI, Dietz WH. Validity of body mass index compared with other body-composition screening indexes for the assessment of body fatness in children and adolescents. American Journal of Clinical Nutrition 2002;7597-985.

2. Garrow JS and Webster J. Quetelet's index (W/H2) as a measure of fatness. International Journal of Obesity 1985;9:147-153.

3. Prentice AM and Jebb SA. Beyond Body Mass Index. Obesity Reviews. 2001 August; 2(3): 141-7.

4. Gallagher D, et al. How useful is BMI for comparison of body fatness across age, sex and ethnic groups? American Journal of Epidemiology 1996; 143:228-239.

5. World Health Organization. Physical status: The use and interpretation of anthropometry. Geneva, Switzerland: World Health Organization 1995. WHO Technical Report Series.

6. www.drweil.com

7. www.CDC.gov

8. www.nhlbisupport.com

9. www.nhlbisupport.com/bmi/bmicalc.htm

10. www.JasonLove.com

11. www.glasbergen.com